Reinventing Medical Practice

Care Delivery that Satisfies
Doctors, Patients and
the Bottom Line

R. Clay Burchell

Howard L. Smith

Neill F. Piland

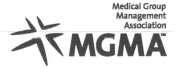

Medical Group
Management
Association

MGMA

Medical Group Management Association
104 Inverness Terrace East
Englewood, CO 80112
(888) 608-5601
Web site: http://www.mgma.com

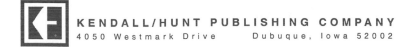

KENDALL/HUNT PUBLISHING COMPANY
4050 Westmark Drive   Dubuque, Iowa 52002

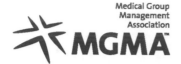

Medical Group
Management
Association

MGMA

Medical Group Management Association (MGMA) publications are intended to provide current and accurate information and are designed to assist readers in becoming more familiar with the subject matter covered. Such publications are distributed with the understanding that MGMA does not render any legal, accounting or other professional advice that may be construed as specifically applicable to individual situations. No representations or warranties are made concerning the application of legal or other principles discussed by the authors to any specific factual situation, nor is any prediction made concerning how any particular judge, government official or other person will interpret or apply such principles. Specific factual situations should be discussed with professional advisors.

Cover photo courtesy of Comstock

Item # 5914

Copyright © 2002 by the Medical Group Management Association

ISBN 1-56829-178-7

Printed in the United States of America
10 9 8 7 6 5 4 3 2 1

Contents

Chapter 1

Medical Groups at the Crossroads

Executive Summary

Medical groups, clinic managers, physicians, medical practice executives, and others associated with the fundamental delivery of health care services confront a tapestry of new realities and causal factors for the health care crisis. Rising costs have only been modestly affected by managed care strategies. As a result, many are looking for new solutions—any glimmer of hope—as a means for addressing the fiscal dilemma in health care.

The structure and process of care delivery have evolved rapidly in profound ways. Traditional premises regarding relationships between patients and physicians are no longer valid, leaving each frustrated and confused. These forces argue persuasively that it is time to reinvent health care.

Group practices and medical clinics have discovered that business as usual is no longer a satisfactory answer. It is time to innovate care delivery by managing four significant imperatives:

1. Reinvent what it means to be a group practice or clinic in terms of customer service, revenue diversification, cost control, and strategic alliances;

2. Deliver productivity from all providers;

3. Intensify medical management without raising administrative costs; and

4. Demonstrate the value of products and services.

High-performing medical groups build effective care delivery strategies upon a solid understanding of the causal factors for the health care crisis and responsive attention to the imperatives for innovating care delivery. This chapter sets the base from which intelligent responses to the causal factors and imperatives can be crafted.

Note: A shortened version of this chapter was published in 1998 as "Medical groups at the crossroads," *Medical Group Management Journal, 45*(1), 62–70.

THE NEW PRACTICE SETTING

"A virtual guarantee of a great return on investment: Seeking investors in a new medical arts building to serve the growing physician community." So read a typical prospectus in the late 1960s, advertising a lucrative opportunity for investors in facilities dedicated to physician practices. It seems like such a distant past these days. Nonetheless, only three decades ago with the introduction of Medicare and Medicaid, the future for physicians was undeniably optimistic and medical practice was a sure-fire financial success. Entrepreneurs tried to capitalize on this situation through diverse strategies offering physicians the clinical support they needed including specialized plant and equipment, medical supplies, office staffing, insurance packages, management support, diagnostic and treatment technology, and other accoutrements of medical care. For the most part, these efforts by entrepreneurs to cash in on medical care were successful, owing largely to cost-based reimbursement, which provided the solid financial foundation for medical practice. Physicians and their practices represented financially low-risk businesses that paid modest attention to office operations. Consequently, investors recognized that their equity could be profitably multiplied by constructing attractive and functionally efficient practice environments such as medical arts buildings.

Fast-forward 30 years. We are in the fabulous Santa Fe confines of Fenn Gallery, a leading art gallery near the world-renowned Canyon Road art colony. This late October day is the essence of Santa Fe. Brilliant blue skies contrast with the glowing yellow-gold of cottonwoods and aspens liberally scattered throughout Santa Fe. The slight brisk tinge to the air invigorates tourists and wanna-be patrons at the Fenn Gallery. The historic adobe building of the Fenn Gallery opens to another world of brilliance and beauty. Room after room of the highest quality Southwestern art is displayed for the delight of connoisseurs. The faint, sweet scent of piñon smoke emitted from classic kiva fireplaces throughout the enclave heightens the experience. Staff at the gallery is discreetly present, waiting to answer your question, cognizant of who really has the means to follow through with an offer.

A middle-aged gentleman sporting loafers, slacks and a blazer is animated as he and his friend examine a stunning painting by Wilson Hurley. A gallery associate moves to within striking range. The Hurley is priced at $80,000; heady stuff for the rest of the customers filing past this monument to nature. Hurley has captured perfectly the play of a fading sunset on clouds over the Rio Grande valley. The fuschia red and soft light of the painting invoke remembrances of Albert Bierstadt's treatment of light. Succumbing to his passion, the gentleman inquires about the price. The associate clears her throat and delivers the steep price tag. Unfazed, the gentleman's response to the associate is confident—I am a physician, I don't think we have to worry about the price. The associate displays a slight, beatific Mona Lisa smile.

Yes, 30 years after the introduction of Medicare and Medicaid, the status of a physician continues to hold sway in many courts. However, by the mid 1980s, the introduction of Medicare's prospective payment system (that is, Diagnosis Related Group reimbursement) began to tarnish the otherwise glossy sheen of the promise associated with medical practice. Within the last 5 to 10 years, many physicians would not so confidently appraise the Wilson Hurley painting for their collections. Many others who are gazing into the crystal ball of the future would forego an acquisition altogether, given the rather somber prognosis for medical practice. The demise of solo practice, the emergence of managed care, networks of care, integrated health delivery systems, cost containment, consumer satisfaction, quality assurance, for-profit organizations, patients' bill of rights and a myriad of related factors have combined to erode the fun, professional fulfillment and financial largesse of medical practice (Azevedo, 1996; Washburn, 1998).

The preceding scenarios and trends have placed physicians (and medical groups) at the crossroads of an uncertain future (Greene, 1996). For many, the loss of solo practice and pressure to consolidate into ever-larger medical groups is serious enough to bring into question the rationale of continuing within the medical profession. The idealized image of a doctor individually caring for patients who appreciate and afford the service is vanishing. The organization of private practice into efficiently functioning medical groups may still remain a favorable context for meeting many professional goals. However, even the group settings have become the target of progressive consolidation and integration. Clinical practice is rapidly losing the qualities and deliverables that encouraged many physicians to enter into medicine in the first place. Instead, providers are discovering a corporate model of care delivery in which physicians have diminishing roles, autonomy, respect, earnings and rewards. The new group practice set-ting does not value the individual practitioner nor the quality of patient relationships. Instead, value is placed on economic objectives that are primarily of interest to an obscure group of investors.

Given that medical groups face the prospects of an increasingly constrained environment and that physicians now practice in settings that are contrary to their values for patient care, and aspirations for professional gain, how can physicians and medical groups position themselves to win in the long run? How can the very fabric of clini-cal care delivery, the medical group practice, and the physicians of which they are comprised, transcend the forces confronting them? How will medical group managers and doctors create a practice set-ting that is consistent with their personal and professional aspira-tions, responsive to economic and financial realities, attuned to prevailing reorganization in the health care delivery system, and sup-portive of meaningful patient-physician relationships? These ques-tions will be answered in the course of this book.

THE PRELUDE TO CHANGE

A Tapestry of New Realities

Health care occupies a pivotal point or watershed in history. Nonetheless, many providers and key players in health delivery tend to ignore the daily growth of the crisis because they are immersed in service delivery. Those who are aware have little notion of what to do about the health care dilemma. Few would argue that we have entered into a period of enormous change—a period in which there seems to be confusion everywhere (Begun & Luke, 2001; Iglehart, 1995). However, despite the prevailing agreement that a serious problem exists, few are prepared to explain the steps needed to set things right. This lack of knowledge about the precise direction in which to head is an ominous prelude to change.

The cost of health care, with its ever-increasing rate of growth and emphasis on delivering the best care, is the most instrumental factor in bringing down the old system (Glouberman & Mintzberg, 2001). Health maintenance organizations (HMOs) emerged as a major play-er in health care and have, to some extent, been able to reduce the cost of care. A dominant and successful strategy by which HMOs were able to lower costs involved substituting outpatient care for inpatient care. The result was a decline in inpatient days delivered to HMO enrollees and, consequently, an ability to lower total costs. With a lower cost structure, HMOs could then provide competitively attractive premiums (Wholey, Christianson, Engberg, & Bryce, 1997). Insights on changes in HMOs are explained in Sidebar 1.1.

Although HMOs represented a new concept in health delivery, they evolved within the old system of providers centered around hospitals, physicians and nonphysician providers or, in other words, the prevailing system of care based on an old set of incentives. The proliferation of HMOs caused new problems due to radically different incentives (Gabel, 1997). One of the ways that HMOs have tended to save money is to require discounts from providers. Providers could either accept the discounts or the HMO would contract with alternate providers. In these market situations, the original providers might lose a sizable portion of their patients if they did not discount their care. Another method HMOs adopted for reducing cost was capitation. The HMO sets a price to be paid for total care for a number of patients. Providers are at risk when complications arise or for more seriously ill patients. These new operating premises deeply affected physicians and their groups because they were accustomed to operating under the traditional set of incentives.

Another crucial indicator of a looming crisis, besides runaway costs, can be observed in the search for solutions. Medical practice is changing so quickly that no one really knows how to respond. In the past, medicine was a cottage industry wherein individual patients selected a personal physician. A referral base had to be built by providing good care over a long period of time. This system had additional built-in safeguards because once the referral pattern was established, physicians discovered that it would be very difficult to lose their entire practice overnight.

HMOs and managed care have altered these facts (Olden, 1996; Tagg, 1995). Because HMOs have thousands of patients, they can decide to contract with one hospital this year and another hospital next year. Thus, a hospital can lose a substantial portion of its patient load if it resists capitation or does not agree to a satisfactory discount on prices. The same is true with physicians. Physicians may not be included in an HMO contract if they fail to deliver the low-cost care demanded by the HMO. The HMO can change contracts, which means it is possible for physicians to have huge additions or losses in their practices overnight. While there is the possibility of an enormous

SIDEBAR 1.1

Changes in HMOs during the 1990s

In a review of HMO growth during the 1990s for KPMG Peat Marwick, Jon Gabel concluded that 10 major transitions were apparent:

1. There was rapid growth of for-profit HMOs and decline in not-for-profit HMOs.

2. A shift occurred from vertically integrated group/staff model HMOs to **virtually integrated** individual practice associations/network models.

3. The growth of mixed-model HMOs (e.g., staff model plus independent practice associations or IPAs) blurred the distinctions in HMO structural characteristics.

4. Product diversification increased:

   - Hybrid health plans (e.g., point-of-service and preferred provider organizations) multiplied.

   - Services outside plans were increasingly covered (to ease choice of plan and transition from indemnity coverage).

   - Administrative-services only plans arose as a means for addressing the complexities associated with managed care.

5. HMO consolidation reduced the number of entities and aggregating population.

6. The decline of community ratings shifted to experience ratings for establishing premiums.

7. Negotiated payment arrangements with physicians became more prevalent.

   - Two-tier and three-tier systems replaced direct payment schemes.

   - There was a rise in capitation.

8. Increased patient cost sharing (for benefits) occurred.

9. Declining hospital use continued.

10. Clinical practice guidelines became widespread within HMOs.

These transitions reflected a dynamic and challenging management environment in which change must be tolerated and, furthermore, embraced. As a whole, this list presents an encompassing perspective on the increas-

continued

ing complexity of managed care. Perhaps Gabel's second point captures this complexity and the attendant challenge best in his implication that managed care groups no longer can rely on one dominant structure. Now they must be comfortable in achieving a virtual reality of relationships; managed care plans and medical groups have entered into a realm where relations are transitory and seldom permanent.

Source: J. Gabel. (1997, May/June). Ten ways HMOs have changed during the 1990s. *Health Affairs, 16*(3), 134–145.

increase in the number of patients in a practice, there is also the possibility of a loss that could financially destroy the practice (Kuttner, 1998a, 1998b).

Patients have responded to many of these changes in medical practice. Years ago, patients chose a physician they liked and trusted. Patients knew their doctors personally and accepted their advice without question. Patients generally did not expect perfect results. Patients assumed they would receive good care and good results (partly because of promises and images conveyed by the medical profession). Patients also assumed they would be treated in a kind manner. Clearly, these premises have changed today. If patients perceive that they have not had good results or were treated unkindly, they sue. Moreover, the other variable in the equation of care delivery, cost, is the one factor patients often use to decide on various options for care. Good care and kindness are more important than cost; but because the first two factors are expected and assumed, cost is the variable that patients typically use to select their provider. Providers often overlook these factors or do not realize that patients just assume they will receive good care. Consequently, providers become angry because their patients seemingly make a choice on cost alone (Buchmueller & Feldstein, 1997).

The Need to Reinvent Health Care

Because the changes confronting health care providers and consumers are so profound, it is easy to understand why trying to solve problems as they arise will not result in a satisfactory, long-term solution. The health care delivery system is beyond improvement; an entirely new system needs to be invented. To do so with any chance of success requires that the basic and unique problems are addressed simultaneously in order to arrive at a comprehensive solution.

First, a major focus must center on cost. In retrospect, the fee-for-service method of paying providers removed almost all restraints on price and, in fact, encouraged doing more than was necessary in an inefficient way. It rewarded extravagance as long as some connection to better care could be made (whether such a connection was true or not). Now cost is particularly crucial because an excellent health care system must deliver correspondingly lower cost. The incentives and rewards today in health care are a direct reversal of the rewards that operated for the past half century; there is little wonder that providers find it difficult to comprehend exactly how best to configure and implement service delivery. Several examples of the adverse impact of these new realities are presented in Sidebar 1.2.

A second significant problem arises because knowledge required to deliver health care has exploded. There is too much knowledge for any single professional to master. Specialties have developed over the years in response to expanding knowledge. Today, from a care delivery perspective, the medical specialties are often uncoordinated and patients have difficulty in reaching the proper specialist. As yet, we have not used effective means to integrate specialties. Nonetheless, a solution can be crafted. For example, the health care delivery system could better utilize progress from the information technology revolution to accomplish more efficacious integration. More intelligent use of specialists would result in a much lower cost, and a better integrated, effective system.

A third problem for solving the health care crisis centers on present approaches to developing solutions. A transcendent solution based on a quantum leap in innovation is needed rather than an incremental solution. When a watershed occurs in business, typically a new, start-up company enters the scene with an invention of the cutting-edge variety. If this new company is really on the right track, it will take over a significant portion of market share as older companies founder. For example, in the steel industry, large, integrated steel manufacturers have lost significant market share to state-of-the-art mini-mills that use cost-efficient electric arc furnaces to produce commodity steel items. Nucor Corporation led a revolution in mini-mills that continues to this day. An agile, innovative corporate culture generated profitability in every quarter of every year in which Nucor followed the mini-mill philosophy. These phenomena of innovation and agility are not always possible in health care because there are too

SIDEBAR 1.2

Adverse Clinical Realities Due to an Emphasis on Lower Costs

The tapestry of new realities suggests that the bottom line (that is, profit) is the cornerstone of what is perceived to be good medical care. For many, this is hard to comprehend and even harder to accept because it is counter to longstanding tradition that health care providers should function like businesses. No present-day health care provider (HMO, hospital, group practice, or physician) can continue to provide care with a negative bottom line no matter how excellent the care delivered. In short, medical care has become a business and most likely will remain a business.

There appears to be two viable solutions: raise charges or reduce costs. It is increasingly apparent that raising charges to produce profit is extraordinarily difficult for a number of reasons. Many larger purchasers of care, such as Medicare and Medicaid, actually tell providers what they will be paid for specific care. Much nongovernmental care is also purchased by large third parties that have considerable leverage because of size. They can demand and receive discounts. They control large groups of patients and specify that providers either meet their price or their patients will be sent elsewhere. It is apparent that the most practical option is to reduce costs. But, even this strategy is complicated as demonstrated in the following three scenarios.

Scenario 1: The Illusion of a Free Market

Recently, a physician moved from a group practice to a private practice. He thought that his practice would be less controlled by administrative decisions and that he could deliver care that was appropriate for patients. To his great surprise, he found that life as an independent practitioner was little different from that as a physician in group practice. He could make his own decisions, but they were virtually controlled by the marketplace. He could perform clinical procedures that he thought were warranted. However, he discovered that his clinical practice decisions might not necessarily be covered by patients' insurance. In the final analysis, he spent the first few weeks of independent practice trying to learn what tests he could order and what he should not do for his patients in order to assure the financial viability of his practice.

continued

Scenario 2: A Policy Dictating Practice Productivity

Consider the plight of the oncologist who specialized in illnesses with poor recovery rates. She spent much of her practice time caring for terminal patients—patients for whom doctors could do little other than give of themselves. She saw near-death patients frequently and spent about 30 minutes with each one, on average, during clinic visits. She was happy with her institution, profession and practice until a new policy was instituted by the HMO in which she was a staff member. This new policy stipulated that terminal patients could not be seen more often than twice a month, and the maximum visit time was to be limited to 10 minutes. Because little could be done for these patients in a clinical sense, the health insurer wanted her to see terminal patients less frequently and for a shorter time. This change would allow her to increase her productivity.

Soon after the policy was instituted, the physician had an appointment with a patient who had become a friend over the course of her illness. They were emotionally close to each other. The doctor did not know how to tell her friend about the new restrictions. The patient came in and the doctor started to describe the new constraints on their clinical relationship. The physician hardly got through the explanation before she started to cry and reached out with open arms for the patient. Both broke down and cried in each other's arms for the next 30 minutes. All in all, the visit occupied about 45 minutes, which seriously violated the new policy and significantly lowered her productivity for the day.

Scenario 3: Dysfunctional Practice Guidelines

At another group practice, an internist discovered that his clinical department had received information about clinical practice guidelines for the future. In the push to encourage the doctors to see more patients, and thus increase profit for the group practice, the historic salary structure would be altered. In the future, doctors' salaries would be determined by how many patient visits they produced. The new guidelines would define an expected number of visits per month. Those physicians who saw more patients (that is, produced more visits) would receive a bonus at the end of the year, and those physicians who had fewer visits would receive a discount from the standard salary. As a part of this plan to increase the gross revenue for the group, internists were encouraged to order more procedures such as X-rays, ultrasounds, colonoscopies and other standard procedures because the remuneration for diagnostic tests was greater than that for time spent with the patient in the office.

The group was paying a bonus for seeing more patients and discounting salaries for doctors who were below the norm in patient visits. The policy encouraged doctors to perform/order more procedures regardless of whether they were medically necessary. This experience enabled

continued

the medical staff to understand the ramifications of clinical practice guidelines. Financially, the medical group had to do something to improve fiscal performance. As a result of the policy, the group was now showing a profit for the owners. From a strictly clinical perspective, the plan had been a mistake and medical staff members were astounded and upset at the results. The physicians realized they were a fundamental part of a strategy that encouraged unnecessary procedures. Perhaps the situation could be corrected by next year's salary plan. The group's intentions had been good, but members had no idea of the consequences when they instituted the policy.

---

many laws, licensing privileges, and regulations that restrict an entirely new effort (that is, one offering an invigorated, fresh approach to service delivery). The implication is that a better solution to the significant problems in health care must come from current providers.

To be successful, the process of reinventing health care delivery requires counterintuitive and nonlinear thinking. This is difficult given the complexity of the current delivery system. It is particularly problematic for those who are entrenched within the old system—a system with enormous, sacred beliefs that comprise the base culture of health and medical care delivery. In building a new vision, creative thinking will have to be used progressively in formulating an alternative scenario. A fundamental difficulty in this process relates to leaving the old model of thinking behind. The challenges for providers and policymakers are to recognize the problem, decide to change, conceive a vision and move nonlinearly and counterintuitively to accomplish the transformation.

Several books have been published about the problems business corporations have encountered and how they must reengineer or reinvent themselves (Hammer, 1996; Hammer & Champy, 1993; Quinn, 1992). The crucial aspects of reengineering are applicable to health care as well as business. With respect to reinventing health care delivery, the first thing is to conceive of a goal or vision of where the system should be at the end point. It is better to be ambitious than conservative about this. This vision is really about inventing what does not exist rather than changing what does exist. The goal of an innovative solution is of crucial importance and must embody the essence or core of what is necessary. For example, the Nordstrom stores have a vision to "respond to unreasonable customer demands." Anyone who has been to a Nordstrom's store can see how well this goal is enacted, which then links with the company's success in retailing.

The information revolution should be acknowledged and incorporated within the fundamental vision of a revolutionary solution at reform. For example, information should be captured only once at the source rather than being collected repeatedly. Thus, a patient's care encounter with a physician at a satellite clinic should be accessible to the system of providers who comprise the care delivery organization. New information is easy to store (in a computer) and transmit as needed, which enhances the health care organization's ability to control costs while assuring quality and accessibility.

Concomitantly, the structural configuration of health care organizations must be improved. For example, departments or units should be combined geographically so that similar units are not replicated at many sites. If customers receive care at several sites, computers and telecommunications should be used to eliminate the need for separate departments. Furthermore, planned coordination should occur to eliminate subsequent integration of separate processes at the end. Controls can be built into the process so that a coordinated endpoint is reached.

The preceding ideas for reinventing health care delivery may seem strange to those who have spent their entire careers in health care. However, new pressures have increased to the point that insurance companies and patients are demanding better, consistent results at lower cost. If these goals are to be realized, we will have to take another look at fundamental operating concepts and see how they can be reinvented to improve health care delivery.

EVOLVING GROUP PRACTICE IMPERATIVES

A Context for Action

Given the tapestry of new realities and the need to reinvent health care, medical groups are discovering that they are at a crossroads with new imperatives. In many respects, there are two choices. Medical groups, their providers, managers and leaders can rise to the challenge of reinventing what it means to deliver care for the 21st century and thereby thrive. Alternatively, group practices can ignore the pressures for change—they can look the other way as the very foundation upon which they are built slowly dissolves, get lost in the rhetoric and philosophical nuances rather than addressing the main issues, or otherwise focus on the wrong variables driving change. The prognosis for survival, much less success, under this approach is questionable.

This book is designed to provide a gentle, but firm, reminder that action is essential for all medical groups. However, it is normally enlightened action that makes the difference between those who succeed and those who fail, or merely survive. In our opinion, informed physicians and medical practice executives are positioned to capitalize on the opportunities that change presents. **Thus, the content of this book emphasizes understanding the context, the pressures that have changed the context, and the desirable adaptive responses that can help medical groups leapfrog over their competition.** By clearly reading and understanding the map of contextual changes, group practices can better negotiate the difficult terrain they face.

Consider the following scenario. An orthopedic surgeon has landed in Albuquerque, N. M., during December on his way to a professional society meeting in Santa Fe. The physician has been looking forward to this trip for some time. Not only is the physician interested in the new technologies introduced at the technical session, but he is also acutely aware of Santa Fe Ski Basin's legendary runs, which have been made that much more attractive due to heavy snowfall. As the surgeon gets into his rental car, he observes that Albuquerque recently has experienced unusual amounts of snow. Should he be concerned? Should he follow the interstate highway? Is the more scenic state route alternative a better bet under the conditions?

The surgeon occupies the position of many medical groups and their physicians. Not understanding the causal factors that can make a drive to Santa Fe a raging terror versus a sheer delight, and not knowing the direction of critical variables (the weather, road conditions) that influence a choice of action, leaves the surgeon in a vulnerable position. The same can be said for medical groups in their naive belief that the present is all that matters—what went before is gone. This is a sure recipe for an unfortunate demise.

Figure 1.1 conveys the challenges looming before medical group practices that must be addressed in order to move confidently toward the new future. The new realities and the pressures to reinvent health care delivery are prime drivers behind this impressive set of expectations that confront medical groups. As Figure 1.1 suggests, the evolving group practice imperatives dictate a set of prime deliverables

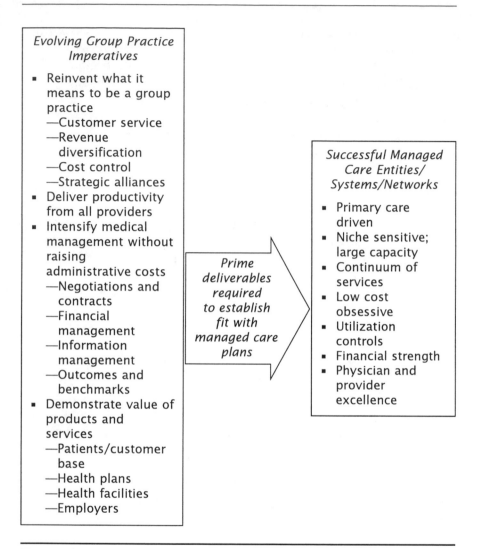

Evolving Group Practice Imperatives

- Reinvent what it means to be a group practice
  —Customer service
  —Revenue diversification
  —Cost control
  —Strategic alliances
- Deliver productivity from all providers
- Intensify medical management without raising administrative costs
  —Negotiations and contracts
  —Financial management
  —Information management
  —Outcomes and benchmarks
- Demonstrate value of products and services
  —Patients/customer base
  —Health plans
  —Health facilities
  —Employers

Prime deliverables required to establish fit with managed care plans

Successful Managed Care Entities/ Systems/Networks

- Primary care driven
- Niche sensitive; large capacity
- Continuum of services
- Low cost obsessive
- Utilization controls
- Financial strength
- Physician and provider excellence

Figure 1.1   Imperatives Group Practices Must Address in Establishing Linkages with Managed Care Plans

required to establish a fit with successful managed care entities, managed care systems or networks of care. Analysis of the health care context suggests that health organizations are rapidly evolving away from an institutional base toward a system composed of networks (Blair & Fottler, 1998). These networks are informal and formal, structured and unstructured, and typically less indelible than long term. The goal for medical groups is to establish effective linkages with a variety of managed care entities.

To think that physicians deliberately attempt to develop close working relationships with insurers and hospitals, even to the point of pursuing these entities, would seem heretical to physicians 10 years ago. However, the rise of managed care and the failure of providers to control costs have reversed the situation. Now, physician groups need to be allied with the very entities they often confronted in the past. Thus, the tapestry of new realities presents an interesting dilemma for physicians. Physicians sense that they are selling out medical care to business-oriented entities; that is, institutions that really do not share the same values, perspective, goals or approaches to care delivery. The predictable result is conflict and resistance because senior physician leadership was socialized under an entirely different context.

For younger physicians, the battle has already been fought and lost. They did not enter their medical education with a view of medicine fabricated around solo or small-group practice. They did not experience professional socialization wherein physicians had almost complete control of operations within hospitals, clinics or other institutions. Young physicians have a more difficult time understanding the perspective espoused by their senior colleagues that medicine and health care should cater to physicians' interests (over other interests). Young physicians less easily recognize and understand that a lucrative income was considered a "given" necessary to maintain physician practices. Senior physicians developed their practices at a time when substantial income was viewed as essential for them to fully direct their attention to care delivery, rather than focusing their attention on the economics of how their practices functioned or prospered.

Young physicians express much less angst about the financial and economic context within which they practice because they have not fully experienced cost-based reimbursement and its few financial controls on the delivery of care. Having already become comfortable (or at peace) with the financially constrained practice environment, they do not have to invest emotionally in the philosophical debate about the demise of physician practice. Young physicians are more prepared to accept the constraints before them and define how their personal practice, professional goals and private aspirations can best be accomplished in the new context.

Although younger physicians are less disturbed by the contemporary medical practice environment, they too are witnessing a revolution in fundamental operating relationships and strategic direction among organizational providers. When coupled with the distress felt by many of their senior colleagues, the result is a less-than-favorable setting for building confidence, trust and loyalty. In fact, these very qualities that have distinguished world-class organizations—confidence, trust and loyalty between employee and organization—are exceptionally difficult to develop when the nature of contractual relationships (that is, managed care contracts) in the health field is one year or less. Consumers/patients are discovering that their relationship to physicians is only as long as their health plan's contract with their employer (Bodenheimer & Sullivan, 1998a, 1998b).

The profile that emerges among junior and senior physicians is not very pretty. Senior physicians are embittered by a radical alteration in their professional practices and, in some cases, their personal lifestyles. Senior physicians have less incentive to fix the system or to work for its improvement as they enter the final stages of their careers. Younger physicians are better positioned philosophically and emotionally to accept the constraints of modern medical practice. They have more incentive to fix the system or otherwise work to improve it because they have decades remaining in their careers. Nonetheless, younger physicians are discovering that they have limited power to affect the direction of the health system, and they are increasingly employees of health care delivery organizations rather than owners. Hence, their power base as physicians has eroded to the point that they are no longer the dominant player, just as group practice faces the prospect of diminished influence within the health field.

Despite these discouraging trends, **the fact remains that physicians and group practices must immediately, cleverly and adroitly respond to the evolving group practice imperatives if they wish to maintain any possibility of exerting influence on the direction of health and medical care.** It is precisely in the strategic adaptations to evolving group practice imperatives that physician groups can construct a basis from which they have higher negotiating power and better prospects of actively determining how they want the health care delivery system to evolve along with their redefined medical practices. In this sense, physicians can remain optimistic because the promise is in the detail. As their practices develop distinctive and efficacious responses to the new imperatives, they will simultaneously position themselves to argue more persuasively for precisely the resources, contracts and affiliations consistent with their aspirations.

Reinvent What It Means to Be a Group Practice

Just as physicians have discovered that what it means to be a physician has changed rather dramatically, so too have group practices realized that they cannot rely on traditional definitions for their identity. Admittedly, this challenge to reinvent what a group practice is known for is little different than the challenge confronting virtually every organization today. Government increasingly finds that it must develop new ways to provide services while its budget is trimmed year after year. Automobile manufacturers have reduced new car introduction cycles precipitously in order to respond to competitive pressures. Sports team franchises are no longer viewed as successful simply because they achieve a winning season. Churches are observing an exodus when they fail to address the expectations of membership for their congregations. Universities are delivering education in innovative electronic and distant modalities in order to remain viable. In short, most organizations today are grappling with revolutionary environments that force them to reinvent themselves.

A leading concern for medical groups is to reinvent customer service. In fact, the very term "customer" is still difficult for many physicians to accept. In the view of senior physicians, the correct term is "patient." They see customers as people who do not necessarily develop a trusting relationship that places their very lives in the hands of physicians. Patients rely completely on the judgment of doctors. Customers may exercise a greater degree of discretion than most traditional physicians prefer. To the contemporary physician and medical group practice manager, the issue of semantics is less relevant than the type of responses that groups are implementing to secure and maintain a customer base.

Customer service has brought a wide range of new approaches to care delivery. Foremost, customer service in small and large medical groups implies a thorough examination, reconfiguration and then monitoring of care delivery processes. Postcare patient follow-up has expanded through survey methodologies including questionnaires, telephone calls and similar tactics designed to achieve continuous quality improvement. Attention to the customer's experience in care delivery and the amenity level surrounding the experience have begun to overshadow the technical aspects of medical care.

The primary point is that medical groups must not only catch up with the rest of the world in how they treat people who receive their services, but they must also envision and then enact how they will remain ahead of other groups in customer service. Fortunately, basics in servicing people remain lead factors in determining success. Courteous, caring and dignified attention to people's needs remains the answer whether for a medical group or a fast-food restaurant. The artistry and creativity in which medical groups design and implement satisfying experiences ultimately explain the differences between the also-rans and the preferred provider.

Revenue diversification is a second ingredient behind reinventing group practices. The traditional revenue sources have effectively redefined themselves. Indemnity plans are now diversified to include wide varieties of managed care options; and, hence, a broad array of payment relationships with providers. The tendency by providers to react substantially in the early stages of diversification among payors has gradually disappeared.

Medical groups only have to look back to hospitals' reactions to prospective payment and diagnosis-related groups (DRGs) to appreciate the need for constructive strategies. When hospitals realized that prospective payment essentially placed a cap on reimbursement, a rush was on to identify new sources of revenue. This strategy resulted in a great many ill-fated efforts to enter promising business lines in which hospitals had no or limited distinctive competence or advantage. The proliferation of health and wellness programs, occupational health services, long-term care and similar initiatives illustrate hospital attempts to diversify revenue. These were the better attempts— many hospitals went crazy in diversifying by purchasing tennis clubs, real estate, restaurants or other business opportunities that appeared to offer a new and better revenue stream. In most cases, these unrelated diversification efforts did little to enhance the operations of the hospitals or the return on invested capital.

The answer for medical groups is to capitalize on what they do best as far as engineering new revenue streams. Unrelated diversification into business enterprises without a distinct linkage to the fundamental services (and products) germane to medical care is questionable. The best answer seems to be found in creating variations of the fundamental care delivery process, as well as the more conservative approach of becoming recognized as the best—the exemplar—in the delivery of specific services. Whichever strategy is selected, the fact remains that medical groups must strengthen their revenue flows through maintaining traditional revenue streams and adding new streams that heretofore were nonexistent.

Reinventing group practice implies adherence to legendary cost control. Hospitals were the first and hardest hit in the pressures emanating from health reform. Their very survival hinged on controlling costs through a very diverse set of players—doctors, technicians, nurses, aides, managers and other staff. Not surprisingly, hospitals discovered that the prevailing incentives did not achieve cost control. Thus began a harrowing battle to control costs before costs controlled them.

Medical groups will continue to replicate many of the tactics and strategies already at play in the hospital sector because most medical groups and their managers have benefited considerably from the lessons learned among hospitals. They also have gained from the general experiences of health care organizations that are emulating businesses in tactical efforts to achieve cost control and better margins. This aspect of reinventing medical groups will continue as groups gain fresh insights on their operations and as they get outside the routine approaches for enhancing service delivery.

Deliver Productivity from All Providers

Medical groups are confronting the cost control challenge in a unique manner as they simultaneously attend to the cost drivers while emphasizing productivity. When it comes to attaining a healthy bottom line, a group practice can raise revenues or control costs and seek greater productivity for a given resource investment. Eventually, the easy cost containment tactics are exhausted and the relative fat in a budget or operation is quickly discarded. It is at that point that the need for real ingenuity sets in and becomes an imperative for reinventing group practice management. The alternative is to raise revenues at a rate faster than costs are increasing. This change can be difficult because many complex variables affect a group's gross revenue.

Productivity enhancements eventually become the tactic of choice for achieving financial margins. Because costs are difficult to lower beyond an irreducible base (that is, there are diminishing returns from cost containment efforts), the group must turn elsewhere for the margin contribution from its set of resources. The answer initially can be found in productivity. If the same (or fewer) staff can produce the same amount (or higher) services without price decreases, then a positive margin can be derived. The issue then distills itself to tactics for raising productivity. Many group practices are not prepared to manage staff or provider productivity as the culture of group practices has typically relied on revenue enhancement of cost-pass-through as the main approach for addressing falling margins.

In many respects, the productivity challenge in groups involves raising expectations as a prelude to change. Until all members of a group understand that there is simply an end to the amount of resources available to run operations, the group is fighting a losing battle. Once staff recognizes that problems are no longer solved by throwing more money at a particular difficulty, the road to enhancing productivity becomes smoother. At that point, the group's management should endeavor to provide staff with the authority and motivation (empowering to design solutions to problems and to instill innovations. The not-so-apparent dilemma for group practices that are earnest about addressing the evolving group practice imperatives is to ensure that all staff members—care providers and support staff alike—are responsible for contributing to higher productivity.

Intensify Medical Management without Higher Costs

The strategies and tactics utilized in productivity analysis and improvement are philosophically linked with another imperative for group practices. Medical groups that are rising to the challenge of the evolving health environment realize that they must intensify medical management without raising administrative costs. In this regard, groups face an uneasy trade-off between heightened managerial control and clinical services control. This tension is an unfortunate by-product of the changed environment—clinical services will not magically become more efficient without analysis and planned change.

The key areas in which groups must intensify their management efforts are well-known—negotiations and contracts, financial management, information management and performance management (that is, outcomes and benchmarks). Every group is facing the prospect of negotiating contractual relationships with managed care providers or networks/systems of care. Because these contracts are normally capitated, groups must eventually experience a gain or loss from their agreements. Astute group managers are armed with information about the cost, price and outcome of their services. Even with the best knowledge, they must be able to drive a hard bargain to the benefit of the group. Poor contracts ultimately spell disaster. Thus, medical groups require managerial skills that formerly were not important in running an efficient and effective medical practice.

Financial management skills have also increased in importance within the last 20 years as far as medical group management is concerned. But, it is only recently that groups are understanding that proficient financial management pertains to a wide array of nonclinical and clinical staff. As financial management skills are embraced by physicians and mid-level and supervisory staff, the potential grows for innovative and comprehensive cost control. More people within the group ultimately understand the variables influencing net revenue and the tactics necessary to drive up margins.

In the same vein, information management is critical for effective, overall management of group practice performance. There are virtually no areas of group performance that are exempt from the critical need for information as a prime performance control driver. Information is knowledge and as a group begins to effectively integrate well-designed database and information system management into its culture, the potential increases for demonstrable gain to be achieved.

Information has a direct linkage with performance management. Thus, quality assurance, quality improvement and total quality management programs depend significantly on the integrity of information systems for their own value. Although most medical groups are cognizant of these imperatives, there is also a tendency for groups to assume that their performance management systems are fully functional.

In the end, medical groups really have little choice but to intensify their management efforts. This statement does not mean that they will spend more resources on management, but rather that all group members, clinical and nonclinical alike, play a critical role in managing operations. Because many providers are not trained in administrative and managerial skills, this presents a distinct dilemma for the enterprising medical group.

Demonstrate Value of Products and Services

The final evolving group practice imperative shown in Figure 1.1 is the need to demonstrate the value of products and services. To some physicians, such a suggestion is hysterical. How could anyone not see the value in the services delivered by a licensed provider? It is not so much that people fail to recognize the general value of health and medical care. Instead, there is the growing importance for medical groups to be able to attract enough market share and gross revenue to remain viable. Consequently, medical groups suddenly find themselves thrust into an unusual environment. For years, physicians avoided any subtle impression that they endorsed or even acknowledged marketing or promotion. Today, they are in the position of having to convince many constituents—through a variety of strategies—that they deliver value for the money; that is, high-quality care for low cost. This challenge is particularly formidable considering the impact of large employers—as customers—in the health care market, as described in Sidebar 1.3.

Patients and customers are more willing to shop for medical and health care services. Twenty years ago, this idea was virtually unheard of as far as patient-physician relations. Today, people are more willing to seek better value for their expenditures and less willing to assume that a single provider is the answer to their care delivery needs. Thus, physicians can no longer assume that patients with even longstanding relationships will remain under their care. Patients are less able to maintain long-term relationships as the amount of health care-per-dollar shrinks. Like other products and services, medical services are gradually being forced into a broad marketplace.

A significant causal factor for heightened market behavior rests with employers. Businesses, which pay the bulk of private insurance coverage, are more willing to shop for the best value in employee health group coverage. Unlike patients, they have little or no emotional tie to a given provider. Instead, businesses approach the health insurance purchase decision from a less impassioned perspective. They want the best quality care, the lowest cost, the greatest access, the most extensive coverage and the least administrative hassle for each dollar expended. Employees want all of these parameters, too, but they also want to retain long-time relationships with their provider of choice. Because the employer normally makes the decision, the result is predictable—corporations make the decision for their employees.

Health plans also play a conspicuous role in the imperative for medical groups to demonstrate the value of services. Health plans seek to enroll the largest number of lives or members with the lowest possible health risk. Employers are the primary target for health plans to

SIDEBAR 1.3

Employer Power in the Health Care Market

The ability of group practices to demonstrate value is integral to their abil ity to thrive in the health care market. By documenting the delivery of high-quality health care at competitive prices, a medical group positions itself to choose which strategic partners—customers—and relationships it will cultivate. In the case of corporations that are seeking to secure excep-tional value for their health care expenditures, the power of the market is sometimes awe-inspiring, as shown in the following example:

> In 1988, the actions of one company sent shock waves throughout the business community. Overnight, Allied-Signal—a corporation dealing in aerospace products, chemicals, and automotive components—canceled the health care arrangements of 80,000 employees and dependents and transferred them into Cigna's HMO plans. In return for this influx of enrollees, Cigna gave the company an excellent price and put a lid on Allied-Signal's health care costs for three years.[1] Allied-Signal saved mil-lions. Its action became a focus of conversation among America's corpo-rate financial officers; the trend of employers' channeling employees into managed care intensified.[2]

Clearly, medical groups that offer value have more opportunities to participate in managed care plans that are significant in the number of lives covered. As this example of Allied-Signal's power demonstrates, not just any managed care plan, or medical group, meets the stringent tests and expectations defined by this large employer. The message from Allied-Signal and other mega-employers is unequivocal—deliver the best health care for the dollar and we will agree to a long-term relationship that also helps you accomplish your goals.[3]

---

[1]A.B. Crenshaw. (1989, January 16–22). Applying the brakes to the runaway costs of medical benefits. *Washington Post* (National Weekly Edition), 18–19.
[2]G. Kramon. (1989, April 18). Controlling costs: One good sign. *New York Times*, C2.
[3]W. A. Zelman. (1996). *The changing health care market: Private ventures, public interests.* San Francisco: Jossey-Bass.

Source: T. Bodenheimer & K. Sullivan. (1998, April 2). How large employers are shaping the health care marketplace: First of two parts. *New England Journal of Medicine, 338*(14), 1004.

attract large populations of healthy individuals. Therefore, health plans must convince employers that the physicians in their network offer value—low cost, high quality, easy access and adaptable coverage for a wide range of needs.

Group practices compete with other physician groups to align themselves with the most desired health plans; that is, the health plans that offer the largest patient volume with the least administrative cost and intrusion on their medical practice patterns. In many areas, the extent of intrusion is considerable if competitors are available. Thus, group practices are forced to make compromises in how care is delivered and the overall standards for serving the patient population. Moreover, medical groups must carefully demonstrate that they can deliver the outcomes desired by the health plans. This perquisite places physician groups in a delicate position of having to carefully manage their care delivery process and the outcomes from care.

The best ways to respond to health plans are through documented quality of care, the ability to deliver a lower price (via cost control), an agreement to provide a range of services in a manner that enhances patient access, a cooperative alliance that builds a seamless delivery system for patients and the ability to contribute to cost containment programs on the part of the insurer. In short, group practices must mimic the shift toward aggressive managed care while preserving the best attributes of socially oriented (that is, not-for-profit) care, as shown in Sidebar 1.4. Documentation does not just suddenly materialize. Outcomes studies are preferred. However, most medical groups are unable to provide the managerial/analytical staffing vitally needed to demonstrate the primary benefits. Medical group management must develop a capacity beyond operations of the clinic. Sophisticated analyses of providers and enlightened cost accounting are required in order to justify the claims being promoted to health insurers.

The Fit with Managed Care Networks

Figure 1.1 indicates that the evolving group practice imperatives define a set of deliverables required from medical groups in order to forge a productive fit with successful managed care entities. In many respects, the deliverables are a necessary precondition for managed

SIDEBAR 1.4

Good HMO, Bad HMO?

In examining the commercialization of prepaid health care, Robert Kuttner has raised the question as to whether all good HMOs must inevitably go bad. In Kuttner's view, there is ample evidence that capitated care delivery tends to bring out the worst in HMOs, but it is unclear whether good HMOs tacitly go bad. He conceptualizes HMOs as either socially oriented or market oriented with the following comparable differences:

Strategies for Achieving Efficiency

Socially Oriented HMOs	*Market-Oriented HMOs*
1. Emphasize prevention;	1. Require physicians to assume financial risk;
2. Pursue cost-effectiveness without relying on incentives; and	2. Require primary physicians to serve as gatekeepers; and
3. Educate physicians in best practices.	3. Select healthy patients carefully (populations/groups).

Kuttner reviews the trends among socially oriented HMOs such as Group Health Cooperative of Puget Sound and Kaiser Permanente. He observes that Group Health Cooperative has made several concessions that mimic market-oriented HMOs such as contracting with hospitals outside the Cooperative, budget leveling, and modifying community ratings for members. In contrast, Kaiser Permanente has suffered several setbacks in the ability to deliver high-quality care and in support from organized labor (notably, nurses). Further, Kaiser is pursuing a national expansion strategy that is often found among market-oriented HMOs.

U.S. Healthcare and Oxford Health Plans are prototypical examples of market-oriented HMOs. Kuttner raises concerns about the extent of risk that physicians must accept if they are to play within the U.S. health care arena—a risk that requires a substantial patient load in order to overcome the law of averages. Oxford Health Plan was the darling of Wall Street until its weak fee-for-services plan inadvertently attracted high-risk patients. The stock ultimately plummeted.

Between these two extremes, Kuttner senses a growing convergence between market-oriented and socially oriented plans. Socially oriented, not for profit plans are increasingly adopting market-oriented strategies in order to survive. For-profit plans are modifying their strategies to be more

continued

attractive to consumers. These strategies are increasingly borrowed from not-for-profit HMOs. The health care market's growing complexity suggests that medical groups cannot afford to adopt a single, doctrinaire position. For-profit and not-for-profit characteristics are increasingly being blended. Medical groups must aspire to incorporate the best practices of both models to become competitively viable.

Source: Adapted from R. Kutttner. (1998, May 21). Must good HMOs go bad? First of two parts. *New England Journal of Medicine, 338*(21), 1558–1639.

care systems or networks. If a medical group is unable to deliver productivity, value, effective management, customer service, cost control and respected strategic alliances, in all likelihood, that medical group is going to have a very difficult time in aligning with the most successful managed care plans.

Another way for medical groups to understand this situation is to consider the characteristics of so-called successful managed care systems. First, managed care systems are primarily care-driven. They must address large numbers of lives—people who need and want the very fundamental primary care services, and who believe that, when needed, they will also receive the best specialty care. If a medical group offers primary care, its goal is to offer better primary care than any other group. If the group emphasizes specialty care, it must demonstrate sensitivity for referral processes and for enhancing the seamless delivery of care (from primary care, to specialty care, to post-care and recovery).

Second, managed care systems and networks are carefully focused on achieving large capacity (to spread financial and medical risk) in an almost obsessive manner, while also tolerating (and encouraging) niche development (Escarce, Shea, & Chen, 1997; Gold, 1997). More than any other parameter contributing to visibility and perceived success, large size plays an important role in the status of managed care networks. The sheer number of lives can help a managed care provider smooth out less-favorable risk statistics over smaller groups of lives among its insureds. A high number of enrollees also functions as a promotional advantage from which informal, word-of-mouth advertising occurs.

Against this backdrop is the managed care system's interest in building distinctive competencies within primary and specialty niches.

Ultimately, people require specialty care. The successful managed care network either provides an array of distinctive specialty services or it maintains affiliations with specialty care providers of indisputable excellence.

Third, the successful managed care system provides a broad continuum of care. In many respects, the system takes on qualities of a vertically integrated system. However, vertical integration simply for the sake of vertical integration does not always lead to the desired goal. Integration must build value and the ability to provide distinctive services across care delivery and patient need areas. Medical groups can develop a productive relationship with large managed care networks by demonstrating how they fill—in a first-rate manner—specific niches in the continuum of care.

Fourth, managed care systems are obsessed with low costs. This characteristic fits in conveniently with the drivers of activity within medical groups. However, because other groups and systems are themselves obsessed with controlling costs, it is very difficult to attain competitive advantage through cost control alone. The strategy for medical groups is to demonstrate the synergy of cost control; that is, the combination of group and system efforts can ultimately achieve economies of control unattainable by either entity alone.

A fifth characteristic of a successful managed care system is linked to obsession with cost control. Utilization controls are impeccable within successful managed care networks. Developing first-rate controls is a very challenging task as, increasingly, managed care networks are comprised of a diverse set of providers, each with a unique approach to quality control. In rare cases, a managed care system may be able to dictate a particular approach to quality assurance. However, the rule tends to be an agglomeration of quality assurance efforts among the network constituents. The implication for medical groups is to develop an uncontested excellence in quality control—a process with demonstrated outcomes that ensures the prospective system(s) will be impressed enough to solidify a relationship.

Financial strength is a hallmark of the most successful managed care plans. Operating capital and capital to finance expansion are prerequisites for large size. The successful managed care entity has deep enough pockets that it is never at the margin of financial capacity. The implication for medical groups is twofold. On the one hand, the group must recognize that the managed care system has more options—options such as hiring its own medical staff if negotiations with physician groups become an obstacle. The managed care network with financial largesse also has the option of weathering the stormy periods—times when competitors try to price-compete or to launch an aggressive promotional campaign in an effort to acquire market share.

Lastly, but probably most importantly, successful managed care systems have built a medical staff of true quality. Physicians and other clinical providers on the medical staffs of successful managed care plans do not just happen to arrive there. A conscious effort is made to bring the best on board and to keep them there.

In sum, many medical group practices must deliver results if they are to align themselves with the most reputable and highly successful managed care networks. If a medical group cannot reinvent itself along the lines of customer service, revenue diversification, cost control or strategic alliances; if it cannot deliver productivity from all providers; if it cannot intensify medical management without raising costs; or if it cannot demonstrate the value of its services, then it is unlikely that it can build an affiliation, or fit, with managed care systems that will contribute to the medical group's long-term viability.

APPLICATIONS FOR MANAGERS

It is clear that medical groups face some very difficult and thorny problems in addressing the evolving group practice imperative and in establishing productive linkages with managed care plans, networks and delivery systems. The purpose of this book is to assist those people associated with medical groups in reading the map of pressures, challenges and constraints as a prelude to formulating successful adaptations to the environment and articulating visions for successful strategies in the future. There is no single, correct adaptation, vision or strategy over the long run. There are only successive distillations of an encompassing vision, that if consistently refined and altered to the demands of the current context, will enable a medical group to satisfactorily resolve the question of approach for achieving excellent response and performance in an otherwise increasingly hostile environment.

An overarching schematic of the path we intend to take in this journey for ascertaining how to build exemplary medical groups is displayed in Figure 1.2. At the heart of the model is a basic assumption that the future can best be addressed if the past history, origins, rituals, ceremonies, relationships, processes and other distinguishing

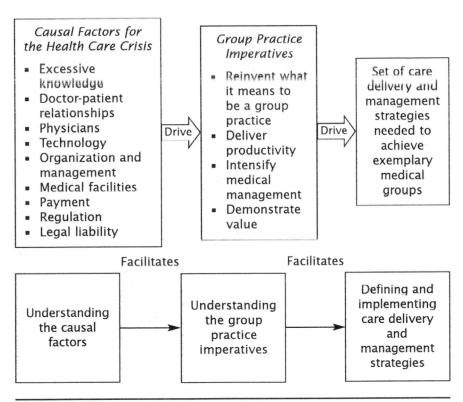

FIGURE 1.2 Building the High-Performing Medical Group

attributes of group practices are honored, embodied and at least reconciled within the transcendent model. Too often those in health care are ready to sprint down the path of action without properly giving time and attention to the essential building blocks that have enabled institutions of care to prevail over the decades. Only an immature view of health care organization and management would impetuously encourage providers and managers to act before contemplating how a new vision or strategy fits within the overall scheme of medical care.

How can a medical group define and implement a set of care delivery and management strategies that enable it to transcend the commonplace answers to the health care environment today and in the future? As Figure 1.2 suggests, before a medical group is able to articulate successful strategies, it should understand two sets of forces—the causal factors for the health care crisis and the evolving imperatives for group practice. The causal factors for the health care crisis include excessive scientific knowledge required for clinical practice, which makes it impossible for any single physician to know everything about care delivery (even in specialty care), diminishing doctor-patient relationships, the redefinition of physicians as professionals, evolution of sophisticated medical technology, intensifying organization and management, the redefinition and reconfiguration of medical facilities, revolution in health care payments and reimbursements, maintenance of regulations and the insidious spread of legal liability. These causal factors drive the evolving group practice imperatives.

As we have seen, the need to reinvent what it means to be a group practice, the challenge to deliver productivity from every provider, the intensification of medical management, and the fundamental requirement to demonstrate value are the manifest pressures that medical groups and their leaders overtly recognize. However, the satisfactory interpretation of these imperatives is explicitly related to understanding the causal factors for the health care crisis. By understanding the causal factors, medical groups will more intelligently understand the group practice imperatives and thereby be positioned to successfully define and implement care delivery and management strategies that address the causal pressures—factors driving the health care crisis and group practice imperatives—rather than the symptoms of those forces.

Medical practice executives can help prepare their organizations to tackle the tough job of developing innovative strategies. First, they can ensure that key individuals who will participate in reformulating and executing strategy—physicians, nonphysician providers, nurses, and support staff—are on the same page relative to the general trends driving change in the health care field. Second, medical group managers should explicitly define the driving forces for change surrounding their specific medical clinics. Clinical and administrative staff should have a crystal-clear understanding of the immediate threats confronting a group practice. Once the general factors for change and the specific threats confronting a medical clinic are known, accepted and analyzed, a promising basis has been built from which creative approaches can emerge that ultimately lead toward high performance.

REFERENCES

Azevedo, D. (1996, August 26). Will the states get tough with HMOs? *Medical Economics*, 172–185.

Begun, J. W., & Luke, R. D. (2001). Factors underlying organizational change in local health care markets, 1982–1995. *Health Care Management Review, 26*(2), 62–72.

Blair, J. D., & Fottler, M. D. (1998). *Strategic leadership for medical groups*. San Francisco: Jossey-Bass.

Bodenheimer, T., & Sullivan, K. (1998a, April 2). How large employers are shaping the health care marketplace. Part I. *New England Journal of Medicine,* (14), 1003–1007.

Bodenheimer, T., & Sullivan, K. (1998b, April 9). How large employers are shaping the health care marketplace. Part II. *New England Journal of Medicine,* (15), 1084–1087.

Buchmueller, T. C., & Feldstein, P. J. (1997). The effect of price on switching among health plans. *Journal of Health Economics, 16,* 231–247.

Crenshaw, A. B. (1989, January 16–22). Applying the brakes to the runaway costs of medical benefits. *The Washington Post* (National Weekly Edition), pp. 18–19.

Escarce, J. J., Shea, J. A., & Chen, W. (1995, November/December). Segmentation of hospital markets: Where do HMO enrollees get care? *Health Affairs, 16*(6), 181–192.

Gabel, J. (1997, May/June). Ten ways HMOs have changed during the 1990s. *Health Affairs, 16*(3), 134–145.

Glouberman, S., & Mintzberg, H. (2001). Managing the care of health and the cure of disease—Part I: Differentiation. *Health Care Management Review, 26*(1), 56–69.

Gold, M. (1997, April 22). Markets and public programs: Insights from Oregon and Tennessee. *Health Policy, Politics and Law,* (2), 633–666.

Greene, B. R. (1996). Understanding the forces driving medical group practice activities: An overview. *Journal of Ambulatory Care Management, 19*(4), 1–3.

Hammer, M. (1996). *Beyond reeingeering*. New York: Harper Business.

Hammer, M., & Champy, J. (1993). *Reengineering the corporation*. New York: Harper Business.

Iglehart, J. K. (1995, Summer). A new era: Modest reform and managed care. *Health Affairs,* 5–6.

Kramon, G. (1989, April 18). Controlling costs: One good sign. *The New York Times,* p. C2.

Kuttner, R. (1998a, May 21). Must good HMOs go bad? The search for checks and balances. Part I. *New England Journal of Medicine, 338*(21), 1558–1563.

Kuttner, R. (1998b, May 28). Must good HMOs go bad? The search for checks and balances. Part II. *New England Journal of Medicine, 338*(22), 1635–1639.

Olden, P. C. (1996, May/June). Managing the managed care market competition. *Medical Group Management Journal,* 15–16, 19–20.

Quinn, J. B. (1992). *Intelligent enterprise.* New York: Free Press.

Tagg, A. J. (1995, February). Prepare now for tomorrow's managed care environment. *Healthcare Financial Management, 49*(2):84–5.

Washburn, E. R. (1998, July/August). Budgeting for a more likely future. *Medical Group Management Journal,* 74–78.

Wholey, D. R., Christianson, J. B., Engberg, J., & Bryce, C. (1997). HMO market structures and performance: 1985–1995. *Health Affairs, 16*(6), 77, 79.

Zelman, W. A. (1996). *The challenging health care market: Private ventures, public interest.* San Francisco: Jossey-Bass.

Chapter 2

Reinventing Health Care and Medical Groups

Executive Summary

The timing could not be more perfect for an enlightened model of health care delivery. The drive for financial success, the rise of anti-managed care legislation, consumer alienation from providers, growing emphasis on quality care to combat malpractice litigation and other factors suggest that the time is ripe for innovation in health care delivery. This chapter presents a compelling vision for reinventing health care delivery that should inspire many medical groups:

> **Quality through the right care at the right time with great kindness and caring at the most effective cost.**

Against the backdrop of the many key transitions and pressures for change in the health care system, this vision provides a logical rationale for service delivery that satisfies providers, patients and the bottom line.

The "right care" implies achieving harmony among cost, provider productivity and physician-patient relations. For many medical groups this idea means more intelligent use of physicians and their judgment In care delivery. The "right time" means that care is synchronized with perceived need and medical appropriateness. "Kindness and caring" suggest carefully configuring delivery systems to listen to and respond to patients as well as carefully enhancing sensitivity to patient needs. The "most effective cost" requires a balance between cost of care and other medical care goals. This vision has the best chance for achievement when patients take an active role and responsibility for their well-being through a personal contract for health.

Five operational pillars are necessary to enact strategies for achieving this vision. Medical groups should create care that is:

1. Physician based;
2. Patient centered;
3. Financially viable;
4. Highest quality; and
5. The result of visionary leadership.

This chapter explains the basis for innovating care delivery through an enlightened vision of medical practice, patient relations and sound organizational management.

A PRELUDE FOR CHANGE

A whole host of issues has combined to generate the health care crisis. Factors such as continuing developments in scientific and clinical knowledge, new assumptions about doctor-patient relationships, redefinition of physician roles, evolving medical technology, the intensifying need for effective management and organizational models, de-emphasis of medical facilities and physical institutions, innovations in payment and reimbursement, the shift away from regulation, and consumer demands for controls on legal liability present a dilemma in health care delivery. However, these very factors, which, in the past, have been instrumental in generating excessive costs, making care inaccessible, creating duplication, and undermining coverage for most people, also represent the basis for a new health system. Granted, in their transitional form, the strategies of health care providers to address the preceding issues have not meshed very well or produced tangible solutions. The profile that emerges is not encouraging due to the range of factors and the difficulty in arriving at solutions that address the pressures comprehensively.

Much of the escalating cost in health care arises from an attempt to patch together a system that is nonfunctional and hopelessly antiquated. An entirely new system must be reengineered, but this system will be difficult to achieve because of past beliefs and vested interests. This chapter focuses on developing solutions that address the causal factors and malfunctions in the health care system. What emerges is an entirely new vision for health care and a startling reinvention of medical groups as a means for delivering care.

Prerequisites for a New Vision of the Best Care

Few people would dispute that the criterion of a good health care system is centered around delivering the best care for the patient. However, evidence is accumulating that in the future, the best patient care will be only one of the objectives of an enlightened health care system (Herzlinger, 1997). It is increasingly apparent that the best patient care will only partially determine what services a patient actually receives. Other considerations include the proper type and amount of care, what the patient wants, what will be legally defensible, and what someone will pay.

The best patient care is difficult to define because medical experts disagree on what is best in any given situation (Ford, Bach, & Fottler,

1997; Jun, Peterson, & Zsidisin, 1998). What is best may not be known, or there may be several solutions of nearly equal value. In some cases, medical experts may simply disagree because of predispositions due to training and experience. Consequently, a patient may or may not receive the best care when all the facts are considered in retrospect. What patients want should be an important determinant of the care received. Many experts on health and medical care disagree about the extent to which patient preferences will ever be a driving factor in determining precisely what care will be received (Donabedian, 1980). However, patient preferences are gradually gaining legitimacy and momentum among providers as a factor influencing the structure and process of care delivery (Kaldenberg & Becker, 1999). This change is in sharp contrast to traditions that accentuated physician prerogative and minimized patient input.

At one time, doctors simply told patients what was good for them and patients did as they were told. Today, more patients want to have input about what is happening in the care they receive (*Newsweek*, 1993). This involvement may work in both a positive and negative sense. Many patients insist on refusing treatment that they do not want. Many patients also want a major voice in what type of care will be performed. Consequently, patients now have far more authority to say what care will be delivered (*Marketing News*, 1992).

The delivery of the best medical care is typically hindered by the current malpractice situation (Crane, 1994). No one can prevent all unintended results; thus, there are cases in which outcomes are unsuccessful. Unfortunately, the legal climate in health care is somewhat different from that of other professions. People who invest money in the stock market and lose cannot sue simply because the investment was a bad decision. There must be proof of incompetence or the intent to harm the investor. In health care, anyone can sue for a bad result. Quite often, plaintiffs win even though doctors did the best they could at the time. Attorneys argue persuasively that, in retrospect, some other clinician would have done better. Malpractice is currently pushing medicine to be more conservative and is having a marked impact on what care is delivered.

Another factor preventing the delivery of the best medical care has been operative for several years. Care hinges increasingly upon reimbursement. If these large managed care organizations with hundreds of thousands of patients decide they will (or will not) reimburse for some medical procedure, treatment, intervention or diagnosis, the end result is that medical practice changes overnight. No longer does the individual physician at the bedside make a decision and implement the treatment. The patient, the lawyer and the insurer become partners with the physician. Any new solution to the health care crisis must take these trends into consideration.

An Opportunity to Reinvent Health Care Delivery

In view of the causal factors driving health care toward excessive costs, inappropriate duplication and incomplete coverage, and considering the many forces preventing the delivery of the best care possible, it is easy to become rather pessimistic about the future of health care. Fortunately, these constraining forces can be overcome if proper alterations are made in the existing health delivery system. Admittedly, bold changes are required. And, many of those individuals and organizations that have previously benefited must recalibrate their expectations. Nonetheless, a reinvented health care system is attainable with the proper alteration of the present system of managed care delivery. Figure 2.1 conveys the essence of a workable plan for instilling innovation and progress that addresses managed care transitions while setting the stage for reinvented health care delivery.

Figure 2.1 summarizes key transitions affecting health care. In the evolution of managed care from the 1980s through the 1990s, a very intense process of maturation occurred. In the early to mid 1980s, the proliferation of HMOs was steadily taking place. Urban settings were especially prominent as locations in which managed care plans could expand. Pockets of the country witnessed startling growth in managed care; notably on the East and West Coasts, and in major cities throughout the Midwest. Nonetheless, many large geographic areas remained without managed care. Small and rural communities did not have the employer base to encourage HMO growth. By the early 1990s, managed care was more pervasively dispersed across the nation. By this point, health insurers and employers were more deeply committed to managed care as a strategy to control health care costs (Hoy, Curtis, & Rice, 1991).

As Figure 2.1 suggests, the ascending spiral of managed care evolution has been accompanied by a number of new pressures. Perhaps most indicative of the transitory nature of the health care system has been the continued search for what constitutes an effective, organized delivery system (Shortell, Gillies, Anderson, Erickson, & Mitchell,

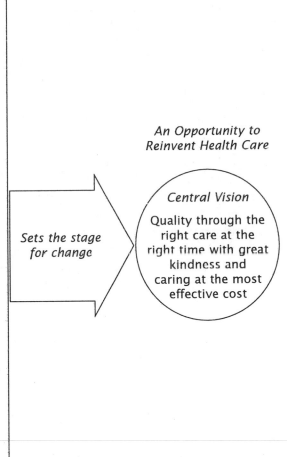

Key Transitions in Managed Health Care

- Continued redefinition of what it means to have an organized delivery system;
- Drive for better organization and management to achieve financial success;
- Shift to emphasis on quality of care (that is, achieving managed care instead of managed cost);
- Rise of antimanaged care legislation;
- Continued consolidation, which drives less choice;
- Patient/consumer alienation from providers;
- Adverse reactions by physicians; and
- Heightened employer efforts to address organizational interests first and employee interests second.

Sets the stage for change

An Opportunity to Reinvent Health Care

Central Vision

Quality through the right care at the right time with great kindness and caring at the most effective cost

FIGURE 2.1   Shortcomings in Health Care Drive Opportunities for Innovation and Progress

1996). Organizational relationships were formerly very structured and seldom violated. Few interactions occurred among competitors or with organizations that appeared to be cooperating with competitors. By the late 1990s, a wave of innovation swept through the field. Delivery systems became based on ever-changing networks, or virtual organizations, that might not exist in following years.

Managed care also stimulated a drive for better organization and management in order to achieve fiscal success (Schneller, 1997). Health care providers have long since grown beyond the effort to work smarter rather than harder. However, the tightening constraints of financial controls continued to demand greater cost control given the stabilization of revenues. With the end of the 1990s, managed care plans became unable to hold down premium increases. The result is a gradual return to inflationary price (that is, insurance premiums) increases that accelerate the demand for fiscal constraint and efficacious management.

Managed care has reached a point that the ability to squeeze margins out of available revenues is an exercise in diminishing returns. Thus, in the late 1990s, managed care providers began to emphasize managing care instead of just managing costs. By managing care within patient populations over a long period of time, there is hope that total costs will decrease, thereby creating better fiscal results.

Aligned with this new perspective is the rise of antimanaged care legislation. Patients and employers are seeking value for their health care expenditures (Eastaugh, 1986). Managed care plans that succeeded in controlling costs without devoting equal attention to the deliverables that employers and consumers seek discovered an interesting backlash (Dolinsky, 1997). Simply cutting back on services and/or denying procedures and treatment has resulted in a new consumerism that demands legislative protection. One example of consumers' reactions to health insurance cost and coverage is seen in Sidebar 2.1.

Managed care in the late 1990s was accompanied by other dysfunctional trends for consumers and patients. Continued consolidation among managed care plans—merger activity among HMOs—produced decreasing choice for consumers. This spreads risk over more members, which stimulates managed care plans' attempts to attain protection by joining forces with other managed care entities. Thus, consumers discovered that although their health care plans were increasingly able to weather the risk associated with disease, fiscal progress came at a significant cost.

As consolidation drives less choice, patients and consumers become more alienated and distant from their providers (John, 1992). There are fewer opportunities to achieve the traditional, idealized relationship with physicians. Physicians observe that the setting is less conducive to their own personal and professional enjoyment. They are more likely to fight the sorts of organizational and managerial

SIDEBAR 2.1

Reactions to Health Costs by Labor Representatives

Fottler, Johnson, McGlown, and Ford (1999) surveyed 205 delegates to the 1993–1994 Alabama AFL-CIO Convention in assessing political attributes of union leaders and members to health insurance trends. The authors argue that organized labor has an important, vested interest in maintaining all benefits, but particularly health insurance coverage. Although the erosion of labor union strength has accelerated in recent years, which raises other issues in priority (such as wage rates), unions still have significant incentive to fight for protection of health care coverage. Union members have traditionally expressed satisfaction with their health benefits. Fottler, et al. (1999) explored the level of satisfaction of union leaders and members with health benefits at a time when corporations are embracing managed care plans in order to control costs.

The findings indicate that union representatives are generally satisfied with their health coverage (note that rounding error is present):

% Satisfied with Coverage

	Excellent	*Good*	*Fair*	*Poor/ None*
Mining and Manufacturing	19	37	25	18
Government and public utilities	7	65	23	5
Services	9	32	50	5
All respondents	16	43	28	14

Only 14 percent of all respondents indicated a critical view of health insurance coverage.

The profile changes dramatically when respondents considered satisfaction with the cost of health insurance coverage:

% Satisfied with Cost of Coverage

	Much Too High	*Too High*	*Fair*	*Too Low/ Much Too Low*
Mining and Manufacturing	15	36	34	15
Government and public utilities	17	41	36	7
Services	33	24	38	5
All respondents	17	35	35	12

continued

Over half of the labor representatives expressed concern that the cost of health insurance coverage is too high. Written comments from the representatives suggested that they wanted some form of national reform to address the problem.

Especially interesting are the representatives' beliefs about the causal factors contributing to excessive health costs (in ranked priority from the factor with highest unnecessary contribution):

- Excessive charges by hospitals;
- Excessive charges by physicians;
- Excessive premiums by insurance companies;
- Excessive paperwork; and
- Malpractice insurance.

These factors have pushed labor representatives to call for national health care reform.

Source: Adapted from M. D. Fottler, R. A. Johnson, K. J. McGlown, & E. W. Ford. (1999). Attitudes of organized labor officials toward health care issues: An exploratory survey of Alabama labor officials. *Health Care Management Review*, *24*(2),71–82.

---

interventions designed to keep the organization and system afloat (Proenca, 1999).

Finally, as suggested in Figure 2.1, managed care has experienced heightened employer efforts to address organizational interests first, and employee interests second. If an employer is willing to continually renegotiate which specific managed care plan delivers care to employees (according to cost and/or quality benchmarks), the employee has a higher probability of being unable to establish a long-term relationship with a physician. The organization benefits because it is able to negotiate a lower cost for health insurance coverage. Patients and providers, however, experience great disruption in their relationships.

Against the backdrop of key transitions in managed care is a window of opportunity. As Figure 2.1 implies, now is the time to reinvent managed care and the health care delivery system. After almost two decades of effort to wring out the promises professed for HMOs and other managed care providers, the sad truth is that the fiscal gains have been modest, and recent health insurance premium increases suggest that the battle for health care cost control was never really won.

The central vision of a functional and reinvented health delivery system is simple. The architecture of a new system should envision **quality through the right care at the right time with great kindness and caring at the most effective cost.** In essence, if, as a nation, we intend to move away from the present malfunctioning health system toward a new vision of care delivery, Figure 2.1 defines the requirements for the desired end result. This is the vision of a system (or the requirements of a system) that is not only achievable, but would create a winning situation for doctors, patients and the bottom line. Each of these aspects in the central vision will be considered separately and then woven together in order to understand the broad ramifications of each.

Many people, especially those involved in health care, will believe that the requirements specified in Figure 2.1 for a new vision of health care delivery are impossible to achieve. Everything suggested may be possible if those in the health care field and the public they serve are able to change their perspective, to see what never has been, and to ask why not? The opportunity for a reinvented health care system is attainable if patients, payers, policymakers and providers embrace an attitude that change can no longer be delayed.

THE RIGHT CARE

The right care—is there only one right approach, treatment, procedure, diagnosis or protocol in the delivery of health and medical care? Physicians have argued that there could not be a single clinical protocol for each medical episode because every patient is unique. Each patient and physician represents a unique individual. In the past, what proved to be best was based on the relationship and interaction between two unique individuals. However, with the explosion of new scientific knowledge in health care and the patient's desire to know more and become more involved in the care process, there are emerging broad definitions of what constitutes the right care. Consider, for example, contemporary physician-patient relations as they exist compared to supportive, patient-care manager relations that can be fostered by any health delivery organization. These two different approaches to care are juxtaposed in Figure 2.2.

Wrong Care	*Right Care*
Contemporary Patient-Physician Relations	*Patient-Case Managers Relations*
Attributes:	*Attributes:*
■ Patient knows their physician at a superficial level. ■ Physicians care for patients as long as possible before referral. ■ Patients are referred to specialists only when absolutely necessary. ■ Patient-physician relationship is shallow. ■ Care instructions are delivered by multiple providers with limited follow-up.	■ Patients know their case managers. ■ Case managers know their patients and their patients' case histories. ■ Case instructions are delivered personally. ■ Case managers facilitate access to physicians and other care providers.
Outcomes	*Outcomes:*
■ Patients have difficulty accessing physicians. ■ Referral is made on the basis of cost rather than on medical judgment. ■ Referrals are less frequent due to expense.	■ Patients have a high level of trust in their physician. ■ Patients can access physicians easily. ■ Patients receive the best care. ■ Referrals are made when medically necessary. ■ Patients are sent to appropriate providers.

FIGURE 2.2 Competing Models of Patient-Provider Relations

Contemporary patient-physician relations are certainly indicative of the wrong care. Patients know their physicians at a superficial level and vice versa. The relationship is best characterized as shallow. There is a contentious claim among physicians that they are carrying excessive patient loads, as suggested in Sidebar 2.2. There are seldom opportunities for either patients or physicians to become familiar with each other as in times past when a close relationship helped with diagnosis and treatment. Furthermore, the current health system

SIDEBAR 2.2

Patient Load Trends among Physicians

There is rampant speculation and many anecdotes suggesting that physician workloads are rising beyond levels that are conducive to quality care and acceptable thresholds for meaningful doctor-patient relations. What is fact and what is fiction given these claims from practitioners? Robert Lowes surveyed several medical groups to shed light on this subject. His findings suggest a pervasive impression among family practitioners that their patient loads are too high and that managed care providers are asking for even higher productivity. Despite these impressions, Lowes did not uncover substantial hard evidence indicating that patient loads have risen as dramatically as verbal claims imply.

A primary point of contention among physicians is the number of patients they must serve per hour. Generalists seem comfortable with a target of serving three patients per hour while specialists have a comfort level when serving less than three patients per hour. The problem as voiced by many physicians in managed care organizations is pressure to serve four patients per hour, a pressure that degrades the ability of doctors to adequately diagnose, treat and support patients. The hard evidence on patient loads does not entirely validate the emotional claims by physicians, as seen in the following statistics. The number of patients seen per hour appears to be holding steady, but the number of patients per physician (in patient panels and patients seen per day) is up.

1993 American Medical Association Data
Patients Seen per Hour

Family Practitioners	3.0
General Internists	2.3

The trend is up:

	Patients per Physician
▪ Patient panel size	1,700–2,000
▪ Group Health Cooperative	1,700
▪ Sharp Rees-Stealy Medical Group	
▪ Patients per day	
▪ Fallon Clinic	25
▪ Sharp Rees-Stealy Medical Group	22–24
▪ Southwest Medical Associates	28–29

continued

What does appear to be changing is the number of patients for whom physicians must manage care. Panels are a convenient mechanism for implementing population-based managed care. Practitioners are better able to keep track of the services they deliver to members of their panel. Whether hypertension control or immunizations, patient panels offer a means for maintaining a discrete patient population. Nonetheless, panel sizes vary according to a number of factors:

Factors Influencing Panel Size

Factors Associated with Lower Panel Size	*Factors Associated with Higher Panel Size*
1. Patients over the age of 65	1. Support from physician extenders
2. Gender (female patients require more time)	2. Low severity of illness
3. Delivery of babies	3. Managed care contract prevalence
4. High percentage of Medicaid patients	
5. Academic duties	

Source: Adapted from R. L. Lowes. (1995, March 27) Are you expected to see too many patients? *Medical Economics* 52–59.

encourages primary care physicians to care for patients as long as possible before referral. Managed care has made it fiscally unsound to refer patients early in their disease episode to specialists. Referral comes only when primary care providers have exhausted their abilities. Care instructions are often delivered by multiple providers—nonphysician providers, nurses, primary care physicians, specialists or other personnel. The outcomes from contemporary patient-physician relations are based on cost instead of medical judgment, reduced frequency of referral (to avoid higher costs associated with specialty care), and access difficulties for patients.

How can a balance be achieved between addressing cost and productivity issues and physician-patient relations? The answer to this question is found in more cost-effective use of physicians while also supporting physician-patient relations through the inclusion of mid-level providers and case managers. A solution that strikes a balance between the excesses of the past and the present is needed for the future.

Physicians and patients can spend more quality time together if physician productivity is raised through the use of nonphysician providers such as nurse practitioners and physician assistants. By providing the bulk of routine primary and palliative care, physician extenders raise the productivity of physicians. This allows more time for physicians to concentrate on difficult diagnoses and treatments. Physicians provide the oversight—close oversight—for nurse practitioners and physician assistants, but they are released from routine care that does not have to be delivered by a physician.

In order for patients to be comfortable with this system, they must be confident that they can access their doctor if severe symptoms continue. Because the physician extender reports directly to the patient's physician, there is implied access. In order for physicians to be comfortable with this system, there must be a ready supply of mid-level personnel who are exceptionally trained and who are interested in collaborating in practice with physicians.

A health delivery system that seeks to deliver the right care might also begin by addressing patient relations through case managers (Freund, Ehrenhaft, & Hackbarth, 1984). A delivery system that is interested in achieving low cost can achieve that goal while also enhancing patient-provider relations (Capitmann, Haskins, & Bernstein, 1986). Physicians should be used in the most productive manner to help control costs and to deliver primary care. However, patients need to have a contact with a provider that they know and a contact who knows them. Case managers can meet these expectations. They are able to invest time in getting to know patients and their patients' case histories. Care instructions can be delivered personally by case managers. Case managers can also facilitate access to physicians and other providers. As a result of these abilities, case managers engender high trust while enhancing access to care. Patients receive the best care because referrals are made when medically necessary. Patients have a better probability of being sent to the appropriate provider.

The right care envisioned in Figure 2.2 is not predicated on a unique relationship between patient and physician. The right care is predicated on the most effective use of physicians and their judgment in care delivery (Unland, 1995). This concept of most effective use is illustrated in disease prevention—annual physical exams. For example, invasive cancer of the cervix can be a preventable disease if women have a yearly cytology smear of the cervix and both doctor and patient respond to the results in an effective manner. Invasive breast cancer is not preventable in all cases but can be materially reduced if all patients have periodic examinations to supplement their own monthly self-examinations and there is an accurate, effective response.

Although every patient is unique as a human with respect to medical problems, the majority of medical cases are not unique. With evolving medical and scientific knowledge, diagnosis and treatment have been rendered increasingly easier through sophisticated tests. Diagnosis has become more a matter of test results and less a matter of judgment. For example, the diagnosis of pregnancy in the first few weeks is very difficult, but with pregnancy tests, virtually no skill or judgment is required. With quantitatively based pregnancy tests, nonphysician providers can ascertain with good accuracy whether or not the pregnancy is thriving. As a result, patients with pelvic pain can be placed in a pregnant or nonpregnant group.

As clinical subgroups are differentiated by testing and examination, the possible diagnoses become clarified—increasingly the right diagnosis depends upon tests rather than judgment. Admittedly, for a few patients, judgment and experience are crucial. However, for efficacy, patients in large, predictable groups (that is, diagnosis made on the basis of tests) should be separated from patients in the small, unpredictable group (that is, still requiring judgment for diagnosis).

There is another aspect of the right care that is contrary to current medical thought but is crucial for a most efficient and effective health care delivery system. Patients seeking medical assistance should see the medical provider with the most expertise. Despite scientific progress, there is still the necessity for experience and judgment in diagnosis and treatment. Maximum expertise should be focused on a problem immediately, not after a number of referrals to ever more experienced specialists. This process means that initial triage would send the patient immediately to the most experienced specialist or subspecialist team. Unfortunately, the existing managed care delivery system presents several obstacles to effective triage.

Primary physicians (and family practice as a specialty) have gradually dominated managed care. This pivotal gatekeeper has provided patients with a contact person in an ever increasingly complicated system. But, as time goes by, some problems are emerging. Theoretically, primary physicians should be able to refer immediately when they believe that more expertise is warranted. Unfortunately, payers are pressuring primary physicians to refer less often. Consequently, there are times when primary physicians would like help, but are pressured financially and through job security not to refer to specialists (Magnus, 1999). Moreover, a referral to a specialist or subspecialist may necessitate several visits when the initial referral could be made on the basis of tests by someone other than a physician. This process suggests the need for a much more efficient triage system where the triage function is totally separated from any medical care junction.

THE RIGHT TIME

The right care must also be delivered at the right time. There are three perspectives for the right time. (1) The time must be right from a medical point of view; (2) the time must be right for the patient; and (3) the time must be right for the system of care providers. The right time is perhaps the simplest to accomplish in the effort to reinvent managed care. The current health delivery system has a long history of meeting the right time in care delivery. Emergencies require the least analysis. They are taken care of immediately, depending upon the condition of the patient. Knowledge of the time limits for conditions are generally known and delays occur only when care providers are overloaded or inaccessible.

In many situations, care does not have to be performed immediately from the clinical point of view. If a patient feels a lump in her breast or has irregular vaginal bleeding, a day or even several days to attain the first appointment does not change her prognosis. Subsequent appointments for further tests or even surgery are often necessary after the initial visit. The only potential danger that patients will not receive an appropriate treatment within the right time from a medical perspective arises in managed care where restrictions (rationing) on care are designed to keep costs down. Doctors may be encouraged to follow protocols for a time period before definitive treatment (for example, surgery) is implemented in order to reduce costs.

From another perspective, however, time is frequently not synchronized with the perceived need. This is consideration of the right time from the patient's perspective and, with respect to quality, it is just as important as the right time medically. There are two aspects here regarding the right time. The first example to consider is the

Care Episode	Care Delivery Response
▪ Patient feels lump in breast	▪ 1–2+ days for first visit
▪ Initial examination recommends tests	▪ 1–2+ days for mammogram and reading
▪ Mammogram suggests cone X-ray of mass	▪ 1–2+ days for specific X-ray and reading
▪ Cone X-ray suggests needle biopsy for definitive diagnosis	▪ 1–2+ days for procedure and reading

Total = 4+ days

FIGURE 2.3   Care Delivery at the Wrong Time and with No Kindness

patient who feels a lump in her breast, as described in Figure 2.3. She calls her provider and is given an appointment in two or three days, has an examination that confirms the mass, and is given an appointment for a mammogram in several days. The mammogram shows a mass and confirms that she needs cone X-ray views of the mass. This procedure is completed two days later. The cone view clearly defines the mass, and a needle biopsy is necessary for a definitive diagnosis. That procedure is scheduled several days later. This time span would not be unusual in our current medical care system and is not necessarily too long from the medical perspective. However, it is too long from the patient's point of view.

When she feels the lump, the patient intuitively concludes that she has breast cancer. Consequently, she needs a final diagnosis as soon as possible. Ideally, this would be 24 to 36 hours after detection. In a quality system, the time frame for diagnosis should not be longer than 48 to 60 hours. The system could be arranged as depicted in Figure 2.4 so that the patient can receive the medical appointment the day she calls (or the next day). The examination is completed, and she has an immediate mammogram that is read instantaneously with cone views taken after the initial reading. The biopsy should be completed the next day and read immediately. Thus, the question (in the mind of the patient) of cancer has a duration of only 36 to 48 hours. After that time, the patient truly knows whether or not she has breast cancer and what the treatment will be. This time schedule is rare in the current medical system. It occurs in only a few clinics where many

Care Episode	Care Delivery Response
■ Patient feels lump in breast	■ Appointment available immediately that day
■ Examination completed and referred for mammogram	■ Mammogram completed same day
■ Mammogram suggests cone X-ray of mass	■ Cone X-ray completed same day
■ Cone X-ray suggests needle biopsy	■ Biopsy completed next day

Total = 24–36 hours

FIGURE 2.4   Care Delivery at the Right Time and with Kindness

patients come for diagnosis. In these situations, the clinics are accustomed to clustering diagnostic tests.

From the patient's point of view, the second aspect of a long time span occurs when the standard of care requires a waiting period of symptomatology to ensure that definitive treatment is really necessary. This might be exemplified by the patient who has increasing problems with irregular vaginal bleeding after she completes childbearing. Endometrial biopsies are necessary to rule out serious illness; treatment consists of hormones or dilatation and curettage. The patient may decide that she would be better off with a hysterectomy to finally solve the problem but may be discouraged because of prejudices against unnecessary hysterectomies or a focus on avoiding major surgery to save money. Ironically, continued visits and tests for the bleeding may, in the long run, be more expensive than the hysterectomy would have been if it had been done earlier. Too often in medicine, little consideration is given to the patient's frustration or anxiety over prolonged diagnostic or treatment plans.

It is evident from these examples that delivering the right care at the right time from the care provider's viewpoint will necessitate some changes in perspective and changes in the way medicine is practiced. From the experience of leading clinics, it is known that short-duration patient work-ups are possible. Furthermore, clinicians have the capacity to provide real-time care delivery. In concept, it is easy to adjust scheduling for last-minute appointments. It requires knowledge about when patients are likely to call (that is, day of the week and month of the year) and when slack time is present in the schedule.

This is a similar situation to that which caused most manufacturers to change from large inventories to just-in-time manufacturing. Initially, no one thought that they would have supplies when they were needed. A perspective change, or paradigm shift, was necessary. For the components that were unpredictable, a small inventory was carried. The crucial change in thinking was that even though some inventory might still be necessary for 10 to 15 percent of the components, it was unnecessary to carry a large inventory for 85 to 90 percent of the components. The manufacturer saved money through reduced storage. Timing was critical, however; and at first there was considerable insecurity on the part of manufacturers. Would each component arrive on time? The just-in-time paradigm shift (in thinking) would probably never have been considered if foreign competitors had not used the new method as a means for manufacturing products at less cost (due to inventory cost savings) and, hence, at lower price. Real-time inventories did work, were less costly than having large inventories, and encouraged people to be more productive. This same type of change must occur in health care if we are to have a productive system.

KINDNESS TO PATIENTS

The third aspect of a quality health care system is that it should be kind to the patient. A kinder, gentler health system should be patient-centered by implementation as well as by pious statement. Several requirements must be fulfilled in attaining this type of delivery system. One is that the system listens to what patients say, with respect to frustrations and attention to problems. This change is easy to implement if consideration is given to solving problems in an effective and productive way. For example, many managed care providers have heard from patients who wanted clinic offices near their homes. Being kind to patients implies careful thinking about how delivery will be configured and perhaps offering superior services at fewer locations rather than mediocre services at many locations. Other aspects of kind care have been identified in research on ambulatory care surgery, as shown in Sidebar 2.3.

SIDEBAR 2.3

Kindness to Patients as a Powerful Care Delivery Objective

Kaldenberg and Becker (1999) studied 275 ambulatory surgery centers across the United States to ascertain patients' satisfaction with the service quality they received. With a large sample of 36,078 respondents, the findings of this study must be given special attention by health care providers. Kaldenberg and Becker sought to identify the factors that would encourage patients to refer their ambulatory surgery experience at a specific surgery center to another person. Satisfied patients often convey positive experiences via word-of-mouth. However, dissatisfied patients typically share this adverse experience with many people.

Kaldenberg and Becker identified the following actors that are determinants of positive, word-of-mouth communications about ambulatory surgery experiences:

- Courtesy of the X-ray technician;
- Courtesy of the ECG technician;
- Friendliness of the nurses;
- Information given by nurses before your procedure;
- Nurses' concern for your comfort after the procedure;
- Nurses' courtesy toward family who accompanied you;
- Instructions given by the staff about how to prepare for your surgery;
- Staff concern not to send you home too soon;
- Friendliness of the physician;
- Anesthesiologist's explanation; and
- Cleanliness of the surgery center.

These findings explicitly underscore the importance of kind care. The primary common denominators associated with a good patient experience in ambulatory surgery are courtesy, friendliness and concern. Note that few aspects of the technical delivery of care are identified as important to a high level of satisfaction. Patients want to experience a kind delivery system.

Source: Adapted from D. O. Kaldenberg & B. W. Becker. (1999). Evaluation of care by ambulatory surgery patients. *Health Care Management Review, 24*(3),73–83.

There are other requirements for a kind system that present a big challenge to providers. Patients prefer to have someone in the system that they know, have met, and who knows them. Patients should be able to contact this provider 24 hours per day, seven days per week, and 365 days per year. Health care systems are enormously complex. Patients seek someone who enables them to get into the system and who then facilitates their movement through the system. Traditionally, this person is their doctor or, by current definition, their primary care physician. The problem is that doctors are not available all the time. If patients need help in the evening or at night, they must use urgent care facilities or the emergency department. Both are expensive and wasteful for many of the problems seen.

MOST EFFECTIVE COST

The fourth consideration in reinventing health care is cost. The time has come when cost must be put in the health care equation and balanced with the other goals. Some will say this is impossible—that a life cannot be considered in terms of cost. Evidence is available that argues for the contrary. Automobile travel is an example. Speed is balanced with safety. If cars could not travel over 20 miles per hour and could withstand a collision of 20 miles per hour, no one would be killed when cars hit a wall or another car. However, a top speed of 20 miles per hour is impractical. The same ends could be accomplished with cars limited to 20 miles per hour and able to withstand a head-on collision with another car. The cars would be like tanks and would be so heavy that they would not offer practical transportation. Cars are made safe and fast, and yet many people are killed in accidents.

The right person needs to perform the right care at the right time. Specifically, doctors should not do what nurses can do. Nurses should not do what receptionists can do. Patients also need a change in perspective and need to pay a premium personally or accept what is necessary for a good result with less regard for the process. Consider the patient whose company was trying to have her switch to a dental HMO. She said she would not change because the HMO dentists had never even looked in her mouth. She wanted personal care by someone who knew her—her private dentist. When asked if she felt that way about all aspects of her life, she replied very emphatically that she did. However, when asked about what automobile she drove, she indicated that she drove a small car rather than a very expensive, heavy car (for example, Mercedes, Cadillac, Rolls Royce). She had overlooked the paradox of her actions. A friend had both a large car and a small car. He took the small car to work one day, was involved in an accident, and was killed. If he had taken the large car, he may not have been injured. The patient was surprised and had never considered that her life and death could be affected by the car she drove.

WITH QUALITY

Nothing in health care is more difficult to achieve at the present than a balance of cost and quality. The concept of quality means something different to each individual. Quality has a different connotation for every patient and provider whether doctor, administrator, nurse, or receptionist. Many people conclude that they know quality when they see it. When physicians are trying to provide quality, how do they decide on a single definition for operational purposes? When patients are trying to choose a health care provider, how do they know about quality prospectively so they can choose correctly? Bringing cost into the equation is just as difficult. Many individuals feel that cost should not be a factor in health care. Whether or not cost should be considered ignores the reality that cost is an important factor now and will be in the future. Either the question of cost will be considered and deliberated to find the best balance between cost and quality, or the system will enter a downward spiral wherein radical cost cutting deletes services with little regard for quality.

In order to reinvent the health care system, attention should be focused on a proper balance between quality and cost as crucial supports of the system. The classical goal of medical practice was to ensure that each patient received the best care. At first, this concept was defined by one physician for one patient. Then, over time, patients began to express their wishes, and patients' ideas became very important in what was viewed as the best care. Sometimes the patient's idea of best care was quite different from the physician's idea. This conflict has been of greater consideration in some specialties such as obstetrics and pediatrics than in others. It has, however, raised the question about who defines the best care. Figure 2.5 provides an insight on how this definition of quality, balanced with cost, might be achieved.

A definition of the best care—or quality care—can be attained through functional teams of providers and, at the same time, the issue of cost can be balanced. The best care requires a multitude of providers—physicians, nurses, technicians and diagnosticians, educators and case managers—working in concert. With the team led by a physician(s), protocols and clinical practice guidelines are defined according to skills needed and according to how providers will work together (Sonnad, 1998; Young, et al., 1997). Each team player will contribute toward the delivery of the best care according to the value that he or she can add. If patient relations can be enhanced via consistent contact with a case manager (that allows the physician to address other clinical cases in order to maximize the productivity of the physician), then the case manager will play a significant role in the delivery of care. The implication from Figure 2.5 is that patients interact with a coordinated, integrated and supportive team focused on delivering the best care at the lowest cost.

As health care has been pondered by various groups, experts and organizations, the term *quality* is replacing the notion of best care. Providers are embracing total quality improvement as the strategy to achieve quality (and, hence, the best) care (Yasin, Czuchry, Jennings, & York, 1999). A quality-centered organization in health care sounds wonderful but, in fact, means no more than saying a medical group will deliver the best care. Quality is a relative term that means something different to everyone. To doctors, it means each can do what she

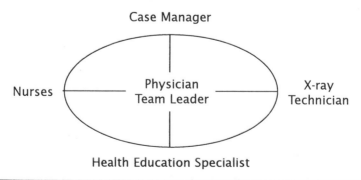

Protocols and clinical practice guidelines are defined by a team of providers chosen according to skills needed and according to how providers will work together.

Case Manager

Nurses

Physician
Team Leader

X-ray
Technician

Health Education Specialist

FIGURE 2.5 Defining Quality Care and Balancing Quality with Cost

or he wants. To a business owner, it means sufficient growth so that the firm can be sold with the owner making a fortune. To a health plan administrator, quality means having the most patients. All large providers now say they not only have high quality for patients, but in fact have the highest quality.

TOWARD A PATIENT CONTRACT FOR HEALTH

It is quite obvious that if the health care system is to reach the quality goal of the right care at the right time with effective cost, patients must understand their own health and become full partners in the effort (Hughes & Larson, 1991). Patients should be well informed about their health status and have sufficient knowledge to make good decisions. This idea suggests that patients receive accurate information and that they are able to internalize this information and, thus, make informed decisions. Some patients will neither be able to nor want to be involved in that level of decision making. Such an eventuality can be accepted if patients realize that because of the options they choose, optimum health care may not be provided at their level of expectation. There should be, in the ideal situation, an informed contract between the provider and the patient about what each can and will do with respect to his or her health care.

Unfortunately, this contract model will require a shift in perspective on the part of both provider and patient. This is similar to the situation with death from violence in the United States today—many people are aware of it. With increased knowledge and medical progress (for example, antibiotics), people have come to believe that if there is an unanticipated result, someone is to blame and that death from illness should not occur. The medical profession has inadvertently fostered these impressions. The result is a belief that care can be managed. This implies strongly that if a patient joins an HMO, his or her health can be maintained regardless of initial health status or what the patient does.

Patients do not have realistic expectations and health care providers do not correct the expectations very satisfactorily. Recently, the concept of informed consent has arisen due to legal liability. The combination of a patient's expectation for success and the doctor's failure to correct the expectation has created many situations in which malpractice is erroneously alleged.

For example, a patient needs an operation. The procedure is suggested by the surgeon. The patient feels success is assured. Success is highly likely, but there can be adverse results. What should be done? To be told that death may result from the operation is not the best preparation for the patient and, yet, death may be possible. It is true that with respect to most operations, the most dangerous thing the patient does the day of surgery is to drive to the hospital. Both patient and doctor may feel that surgical success is highly likely, but neither may have true perspective or understanding that medical care is usually choosing the better or best of several bad alternatives. A more realistic perspective is presented in Figure 2.6 wherein the patient realizes that some alternatives are better than others. The best choice is often based on what the patient needs with respect to living. Is it better to put up with gallbladder attacks or to have an operation that will almost certainly solve the problem but carries a significant increase in short-term risk?

If the health care system could alter patients' perspective about their own mortality, then risks and results of treatments could be considered. Helping patients to acquire accurate knowledge and perspective about health has been brought into focus by legal liability and malpractice actions (Hickson, Clayton, Githens, & Sloan, 1992). Informing patients is one strategy to minimize malpractice litigation.

- Patients receive accurate substantive information about the diagnosis, prescribed treatment and prognosis.
- Options for treatment are defined.
- Probable results from treatment are explained.
- Lifestyle impact from treatment is discussed.
- Patient responsibilities are identified.

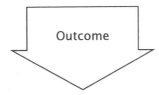

Outcome

Patient becomes an integral part of case delivery.

FIGURE 2.6   Personal Contract for Health Under Conditions of Impending Surgical Procedure

In the final analysis, information is most crucial for moral and ethical reasons. Patients should understand and be able to make informed decisions even if it is difficult (Pontes & Pontes, 1997).

With respect to health maintenance, patients should be expected to do some things in assuming responsibility for their health. Yet, for the most part, many do not do so even though informed. That is why there should be a personal contract with each patient.

Pregnancy is an example in which expectations are often unrealistic. Pregnancy is safe and good results for mother and baby are usually achieved. However, some studies have shown that when a woman becomes pregnant, her chances of dying within the next 12 months are increased by a factor of 10. Granted, the risk of death is very small and the rewards of a successful pregnancy are enormous, but in almost all other situations, human beings would think carefully about choosing one of two paths that increase their potential mortality by a factor of 10. The result is that some women consider pregnancy without any regard to lifestyle changes and most health care providers are totally optimistic about perfect results. The provider-patient interaction gives the strong impression that results will be positive. When they are not, there is consternation. A more realistic preparation of the patient by the physician would entail communicating that getting pregnant is a serious matter; it is quite safe, but certainly more risky than not being pregnant. Providers will do their best to ensure a good outcome for both mother and baby, but success cannot be guaranteed.

To achieve a realistic intervention between providers and patients will require a number of important changes. For example, HMOs can alter their approach to marketing and promotion. Instead of communicating that they provide the best care, HMOs can become more responsible in defining their product, describing the ways in which they prevent rationing, how they reduce costs, and what they expect of patients. This may seem contradictory from a promotion and marketing viewpoint, but evidence is accumulating that malpractice and legal liability are so serious that no one who expects to remain in health care would consciously want to enroll anyone under the slightest false pretense. Thus, an intelligent marketing program would define the product, have clear deliverables, never promise what it cannot deliver, and ideally deliver more than promised.

A personal contract for each patient is crucial upon entry into the system, as shown in Figure 2.7. The health of each patient should be

- On entry into a managed care plan, each patient has a complete health assessment.
- Assessment team identifies risk factors and proposes a plan for interventions and lifestyle changes.
- Patient and care team sign a contract for managing care.
- As health milestones are reached, patient's premiums are lowered.

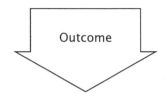

Outcome

Patient has a direct, financial incentive
to become an integral part of care delivery.

FIGURE 2.7 Personal Contract for Health under Managed Care

evaluated in depth and discussed with the patient by the case manager. There is enormous difference between healthy and nonhealthy patients. Too often, patients are considered the same regardless of health, exercise or ability to promote their own health. Then, once in the system, if patients have a heart attack, their illness is considered differently. It would be far better to consider each patient individually upon entry.

After evaluation and discussion, it should be clear to the patient what the providers suggest in order to treat a malady. Similarly, what the patient should do in response should also be clear. Providers will then find out realistically what the patient can and will do. The patient's inability to do what is best should not be glossed over or changed by coercion. This contract will alter the legal liability and, in the future, might alter the price paid for the health care. Should someone aged 50 who smokes more than 50 cigarettes a day pay the same for health care as someone who does not smoke at all? If there is a differential cost, it should only be with respect to actions the patient has some control over and not merely with the current health status that is involuntary. A price differential with regard to voluntary actions might help patients alter behavior in a health-promoting direction.

The concept of case managers and expert teams providing patient care provides a background and infrastructure for realistic expectations, informed care and intelligent decision making (Liedtka & Whitten, 1998). The case manager has the time to discuss health status in detail after the thorough health evaluation by the team. The case manager can find out what the patient expects of the system and what he or she is able to do in taking responsibility. What is most desirable is clear, and there are defined boundaries. The contract can be signed and the case manager can endeavor to make certain that it is adhered to by both parties (or modified). As a result of the specific contract, the probable end results can be anticipated and discussed.

With respect to the risk of procedures, it is important that the provider performing a procedure be included in the plan to inform the patient. However, it is often better for the patient to be informed of risks by another team member such as the case manager. Under the current system of care delivery, a surgeon may have to suggest the operation, describe why it is necessary, and then (for purposes of informed consent) discuss the dangers. In a reinvented health care system, the case manager, or another member of the team, could more easily and effectively ensure that the patient had realistic expectations about indications, success rates and dangers of a procedure.

STRATEGIES FOR REINVENTING MEDICAL GROUPS

Just as the health care system can only be reformed if an entirely new way of thinking is incorporated in its redesign, so too must a fresh approach be taken in the revitalization of medical groups. While health care policymakers have enormous influence on the ultimate reimbursement incentives that drive providers, and while the public debate captures attention concerning the directions health policy might take, the true ability to reinvent the health delivery system is found at the level of providers. Medical groups represent the common denominator from which health reform will be articulated. Medical groups and their clinical context offer the bridge to patients. Medical groups and the care they deliver effectively provide a realistic translation to patients, making health care tangible and the delivery experience a blessing or a curse. Consequently, if an answer is going to be found and acted upon, the most likely setting in which change will occur is among medical group and clinics.

Medical groups essentially represent the point at which maximum constraints on change may be found. The setting in which most physicians and support staff practice is also the context that ultimately determines whether the far-reaching aspirations of a more functional and cost-effective health care system are attained (Kralewski, Wingert, & Barbouche, 1996). After all of the philosophizing by health care experts has waned; after all of the politically correct statements about health reform have been uttered by politicians; after all of the self-interests of physicians, nurses, therapists, lawyers, administrators and others with a vested link to care delivery have been expressed, it is still the practitioner working with the patient who will essentially enact any fundamental improvements, or reinvention, in the delivery system.

If this argument is accepted, then the issue really distills to determining how medical groups can evolve in very practical terms to make innovation and reform a reality. How can a new approach to care delivery be operationalized? How can a fundamentally improved philosophy of care delivery be implemented? How can providers be more effectively orchestrated to produce functional teams wherein provider and patient goals are consonant and care delivery attains ends that are mutually desired? How can reform be initiated at the grass-roots level without involving enormous budgets and without political compromises? How can medical groups reach the forefront of reform and, in the process, become the role model for an enlightened health care delivery system? These questions will be answered in the remainder of this book.

An overview of our vision is shown in Figure 2.8, which displays the goals that exemplary medical groups seek to achieve—the same goals necessary to reinvent health care delivery—along with five operational pillars for medical groups. The operational pillars provide the specific strategies and actions whereby high-performing medical groups can achieve the right care at the right time with kindness, low cost and quality. Each of the operational pillars will be discussed at length throughout this text. For the moment, it is appropriate to consider that by carefully instilling a new philosophy, principles and methods of operating—physician-based, patient-centered, financially viable, highest quality and visionary leadership—medical groups can lead a revolution. These operating principles translate into mechanisms for achieving a fundamentally improved vision of health care delivery. We maintain that providers—in particular, physicians—can exercise proper leadership in their practices to achieve what politicians and policymakers have been unable to achieve over the last 30

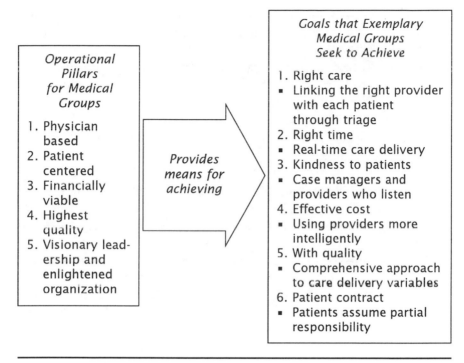

FIGURE 2.8 Operational Pillars that Assist in Reinventing Medical Groups

years. Physicians can provide the leadership necessary to create a revolution in the health care system—a revolution that centers in medical groups and clinical settings.

Five Operational Pillars Underlying a Dramatic Evolution

Five pillars support a dramatic evaluation of health care and, in turn, define an agenda of action for exemplary medical groups. First, and foremost, if any progress is to be made in reinventing health and medical care delivery, then solid solutions will center around physicians (see Chapter 3). Only a physician-based system has promise for rectifying the problems that beset health care delivery (Succi & Alexander, 1999). In the final analysis, it is the clinician who helps people overcome disease. Patients recognize this and will act aggressively to ensure that they have access to providers they are comfortable with and trust. Yet, much of the rhetoric surrounding health policy implies that physicians and valuable patient-physician relationships can be discounted in the effort to achieve health reform. In our view, successful reinvention of health care delivery begins by honoring the centrality of physicians and patient-physician relations. Physician-based reengineering of health care delivery presents a foundation from which significant change and progress can be made. However, physicians face several obstacles that limit their ability to contribute effectively to change.

Figure 2.9 presents an overview of several of the significant constraints on physicians. Administrative interventions implemented by many managed care plans have sought to control the cost of care and, secondarily, to address quality. Primary care gatekeeping, utilization management, practice guidelines, physician profiling and focused studies of quality of care have been imposed by most managed care plans. In other cases, managed care plans have introduced risk sharing (that is, placing physicians at financial risk on a partial or complete capitation basis for care to a cohort of patients). Accompanying these impositions, many institutional providers have controlled resource support available to physicians in scheduling suites for surgical procedures, in access to diagnostic and treatment equipment and in support staffing.

The culmination of organizational and managerial constraints by medical groups and managed care plans on physicians is a decided disconnect with the professional who can do the most to help lower costs and improve quality. A coercive approach to physician relations will do little to make progress toward cost containment and quality enhancement goals that are dominating the health care debate. Chapter 3 defines several successful strategies for incorporating physicians in a constructive way while simultaneously achieving an improved health care system.

A second important pillar in reinventing medical groups relates to patients. If physicians represent the primary reason for a medical group's existence, then patients are the ultimate reason why medical groups offer services. High-performing medical groups are those that attend to the needs of their customer base—patients. Medical groups must forge a stronger connection with their clientele. It is unlikely that an effective managed care strategy can be implemented unless those who deliver the care and those that receive the care are closely connected and in harmony.

Organizational Constraints on Physicians

Administrative interventions:

- Gatekeeping of referrals;
- Utilization management;
- Practice guidelines;
- Physician profiling; and
- Focused studies of quality of care.

Financial incentives:

- Risk sharing (partial or complete capitation)

Conditions of Work:

- Resource support to practice

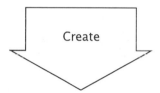

Coercive approach to solving health care delivery issues

FIGURE 2.9 The Unintended Consequences of Physician Management

Source: Adapted from D. Blumenthal. (1996). Effects of market reforms on doctors and their patients. *Health Affairs, 15*(2): 170–184.

There are many reasons to believe that physicians and patients are seriously disconnected from one another. Figure 2.10 conveys the erosion of patients' trust in physicians that is occurring due to how managed care plans and medical groups structure care. Utilization review and other organizational constraints, such as profiling and gatekeeping, act as dampers on how physicians practice (Lagoe & Aspling, 1996). Physicians are restricted from referring patients to the specialists they want to access. Physician panels restrict patient choice of provider. Utilization management may create contradictory messages regarding what treatment will be versus what is desired. Confusion surfaces regarding who actually is in control of care delivery. In extremes, clinical policies control what information may be shared with patients.

Utilization review and structural arrangements (for example, gatekeeping roles) potentially challenge trust in physicians by:

- Restricting choice;
- Contradicting medical decisions;
- Confusing control of care delivery; and
- Restricting open communication with patients.

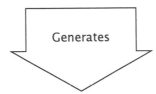

Generates

Disconnection between provider and patient

FIGURE 2.10   The Erosion of Patients' Trust in Physicians

Source: Adapted from D. Mechanic & M. Schlesinger. (1996, June 5). The impact of managed care on patients' trust in medical care and their physicians. *JAMA.* *275*(21): 1693–7.

The culmination of the trends toward managed care is quite simple. Many patients no longer trust physicians, the managed care plans for which physicians perform services and the medical groups in which physicians work. Thus, high-performing medical groups will reestablish trust with their clients, patients and consumers as a first step toward reinventing medical practice. The equation must balance physician and patient. Chapter 4 presents many promising strategies for reconnecting with patients and establishing a balance between physician and patient goals.

The third pillar states that medical groups must take the lead in cost control as a means to create financial viability for themselves and the health care system (see Chapter 5). To this point in the evolution of health care delivery, physicians and other providers have reacted to reimbursement policies as a means for ensuring their own well-being. The result has been a strategic battle wherein physicians have tried to reconfigure their service delivery patterns to obtain optimal payment and the best return on investment for patient care. A driving motivation has been economic self-interest, although many physicians would argue otherwise. There is nothing wrong with looking out for one's self-interest except when the consequences of that behavior threaten the very well-being of the health delivery system. Another approach is possible. Physicians can begin to think of patient care delivery from the perspective of how they assure patient well-being as well as how physicians can assure their own economic well-being.

The ability to achieve financial viability entails not only intensive and far-reaching efforts to contain the actual costs of producing care, but also efforts at making all health care resources more productive, especially physician inputs to the delivery process. The problem in controlling costs is the erroneous perception by many that the fat has been cut from the care delivery process. Not enough effort has been made to reengineer care delivery in a manner that truly seeks to control costs without sacrificing quality. Substantial gains at cost savings are possible, but not if we continue to provide care in the same manner that physicians have practiced over the decades. A paradigm shift in delivery is the most promising tactic for arriving at further cost containment gains.

Productivity management is an attendant tactic that can be implemented with cost containment efforts. A wide variety of approaches exists, including team-based, patient-centered, procedural, facility-based and personnel strategies (Trey, 1996). However, as with cost containment, the initial thrust should be a paradigm shift in thinking that discards the traditional assumptions and substitutes innovative tactics that focus on creativity rather than traditions and rituals. Although productivity enhancement is not a cure-all, it offers particular promise in the group practice setting where provider roles have become ingrained to the detriment of optimal resource use. Many aspects of health care delivery contribute to rising costs, especially factors that are beyond the control of physicians. For example, the care delivery benefit of new medical technology, the physiologic responses of the human body, and the patient's contribution to maintaining health and pursuing recovery are a few of the uncontrolled variables (as far as physicians are concerned) that raise costs. Nonetheless, in the medical group practice setting, physicians can control how they organize care delivery and, hence, affect not only their own productivity but the cost of care as well.

Chapter 5 introduces the concepts of medical manufacturing, an effort by medical groups to embrace ideas from corporate and industrial settings that have been proven to enhance productivity. The goal-focused medical group discards the time-honored structure and process of care delivery in favor of analyzing the optimal delivery process, a process that centers on end results rather than prerequisites and traditions (Lowes, 1998). Sidebar 2.4 provides an example of medical manufacturing for an influenza outbreak. There is every reason to believe that emerging medical professionals are less bound to the traditions of medical care than were their predecessors. As a result, there is a greater probability that medical groups in the future will be able to adopt corporate techniques associated with the delivery of services.

The fourth pillar, discussed in Chapter 6, is the delivery of high quality care. Not only are medical groups challenged to instill quality within care delivery processes, but they also face the pressures of limiting litigation. When quality improvement strategies are applied consistently, medical groups can attain higher patient satisfaction and lower malpractice litigation. The key is in effective patient communication and integrating case managers within the care delivery process. The ability of medical groups to incorporate patients within the process for limiting liability is another overlooked strategy. Too often provider groups view litigation prevention as a responsibility for practitioners within the group. By integrating patients, a much more effective process unfolds with significant promise for reduced litigation. Medical groups at the cutting edge of care delivery construct quality assurance processes throughout the service delivery effort, and then utilize the information from quality improvement processes to enact constructive changes—changes that go beyond the surface of care to include the redesign of service delivery as indicated.

The final pillar for medical groups that are pursuing efforts to reinvent health care includes visionary leadership and enlightened organization (see Chapter 7). For decades, administration, management and leadership have been viewed by physicians in an adversarial way. Management has been a convenient scapegoat for physicians and other clinicians to explain why medical practice has become such a nonattractive professional setting. Physicians and other providers can either continue believing this myth or they can respond constructively by actively participating in the leadership and management of their group practices. The high-performing medical group originates from physicians who participate in their administrative and organization structure, who assume leadership positions not just for the sake of control but to instill the best system of managing care delivery (Goes & Zhan, 1995). Granted, most physicians did not enter

SIDEBAR 2.4

Medical Manufacturing and an Influenza Outbreak

Every year the public is at risk for an influenza outbreak. Managed care plans exhort the virtues of receiving a flu shot in order to prevent contagion or to minimize the adverse effects if a person does become contaminated. When the flu outbreak arrives in a community, what is the typical reaction by the health care community? Usually, there are a series of health education promotions on differentiating between the flu and a common cold. Instruction is conveyed on symptoms that suggest when a visit to the doctor is appropriate. Beyond these reactions, the delivery system barely responds. Patients who contract the flu try to see their physicians. The medical providers are overwhelmed because their caseload has risen dramatically with many people who have the same or similar symptoms. This leaves less time for those with other, serious problems.

A managed care plan that aspires to improve its service delivery, while controlling cost and raising quality, should consider a temporary team assigned to the flu outbreak. That team could be comprised of several nurse practitioners and a physician who have the primary responsibility of diagnosing and treating flu symptoms. Patients who call for an appointment with their regular physician might have several days to a week before they can obtain an appointment. However, with the special flu team, they can receive an appointment that very day. If, in the course of being diagnosed by the nurse practitioner, a patient displays symptoms that are not flu-like, the patient can be referred to the physician providing oversight to further diagnose the patient's problem. A case manager is available to enable that patient to negotiate the system for further referral or diagnosis and treatment.

In the preceding scenario, it makes more sense from fiscal and medical practice perspectives to form a temporary team to address an outbreak of the flu. Patients are generally cognizant of what is happening around them. They know if their co-workers or friends are reporting experiences with the flu. When they experience similar symptoms that do not improve and that may indicate more serious illness (for example, pneumonia), they do not necessarily have to see their personal physician—particularly if it will require several days to see that specific doctor. They may seek an examination to determine that they do not have initial stages of pneumonia or they may seek antibiotics. The point is that they

continued

do not necessarily have to see their physician, nor do they want to put up with the hassle of trying to see that physician who is already booked with too many patients manifesting similar symptoms. By developing a systematic, problem-oriented approach to a morbidity outbreak, the managed care plan keeps costs down and assures quality while also maintaining desirable patient relations.

---

medicine to become managers, but until they recognize that managing is an integral part of care delivery, physicians will continue to relinquish control to nonphysicians (Davidson, McCollom, & Heineke, 1996).

THE VISION REALIZED

Let us examine the results from applying the five operational pillars in a hypothetical medical group. Assume that the group commits itself to using physicians as a means to control costs. In the initial phase, the group adopts the philosophy that physicians can be extended through mid-level providers (Meighan, 1995). This strategy enables the group to lower costs, to raise physician productivity and to build better bridges to patients. Obviously, not every medical group can adopt mid-level providers as a feasible operating tactic nor can every group agree that this approach to care delivery is desired. The point is that innovative rethinking of how to control costs and raise productivity can eventually help achieve the goals of transcendent health care.

As an additional effort to improve service delivery, assume that the medical group contemplates approaches at medical manufacturing to enhance provider productivity. The group introduces a triage team to better link patients with the correct provider (Liedtka & Whitten, 1997). The triage team must act decisively and swiftly to prevent becoming a bottleneck in the delivery of care. By assessing patient needs and provider capabilities, the triage team is better able to match patients directly to the appropriate care providers, thus focusing the right care on the right patient at the right time and avoiding duplicative care by the wrong providers. Again, the goals of improved health care delivery are achieved—the right care is accomplished at the right time with effective cost.

The medical group may seek further improvements in its quest. Assume the group adopts a team of case managers who participate on the triage team. The case managers are retained for their ability to listen carefully to patients and to communicate patient concerns/issues/questions and other expectations to providers (Lowes, 1996). The case managers demonstrate an uncanny ability to translate patient perceptions and desires into an understandable parameter of health care delivery. The result is more satisfied patients who know what will be done to them and why and the result is a care delivery process that adapts itself to the individual needs of each patient. These operating pillars help the medical group to deliver the right care at the right time with great kindness and quality. Patients are less likely to institute malpractice litigation because they have been consulted and ultimately integrated in the care delivery process in a nonsuperficial fashion.

Not content with the advances it has achieved by altering medical care delivery, the medical group goes another step by preparing a written patient contract for care. Patients are educated about the medical group's philosophy that patients have a responsibility to maintain their health and to assist in the process of recovering from episodes of care. The medical group launches a continuous health promotion program via newsletters and counseling (through the case managers) that continually reinforces the philosophy. The result is a marked decrease in patients' complaints about their recovery, shortened recovery times, and fewer visits for noninvasive procedures. The group discovers that its experience rating is dramatically improved. As a result, the group is able to contract with a managed care plan to provide coverage over an entirely new set of lives (that is, patients). Thus, the group has been able to provide documented quality of care wherein each patient's contract for responsibility has assisted provider efforts.

Finally, assume that the medical group throws out its traditional hierarchy of authority and moves toward teams in managing its operations. The initial short-run is disconcerting and staff members tend to fight the ambiguity of the situation. However, before long, physicians, nurses and case managers notice that they are better able to treat the entire patient, rather than parts of patients. Furthermore, they discover that they are better able to incorporate staff from the business office in monitoring the cost of care options. The result is more effective cost with quality.

These illustrations of strategies adopted by the hypothetical medical group may not work perfectly for all providers. However, the point of the illustrations is that the willingness to innovate—to think out of the box—can start a group down the path toward enlightened health care delivery. By shifting the paradigm of thinking about how medical providers should function and how patients should be involved in the care delivery process, medical groups can overcome the realities of care delivery. They can transcend the self-imposed constraints about the true possibilities of care. They can move beyond the status quo in reaching the point where they are performing the right care at the right time with kindness to patients at effective cost and with high quality.

APPLICATIONS FOR MANAGERS

The vision of quality through the right care at the right time with kindness and care at most effective cost based upon a patient contract of responsibility is a lofty reach for many medical groups. It is too easy to argue that the current system is excessively cumbersome and unsupportive of change, or that many of the factors in the equation represented by the vision are not controllable by any one medical group. As long as medical groups, their providers and managers think in this fashion, it is certain that an inspirational vision—any stretch of aspirations—will never be attained.

The vision espoused in this chapter presents a concept that medical groups can use as a draft template. The process of innovating care delivery requires bold ideas and courageous actions. It is most probable that medical groups interested in moving toward more enlightened service delivery can use this vision as a starting point for refining a unique and individualistic concept of their own. In this respect, the implications of this chapter for the typical medical group are numerous. **A vision must be created that guides the formation and execution of strategies—strategies that lead to solutions rather than the perpetuation of problems.**

Of course, there is risk in moving out ahead from the mass of medical groups who linger in complacency, befuddled by the conflicting messages they receive from their many internal and external stakeholders. It is possible that a medical group will articulate an incorrect vision. The group's team of providers, managers and patients may reach beyond their resources and capabilities. They may define an inspiring and effective vision, but execution of specific tactics may cause problems. In short, there is no guarantee that stepping out with a bold conception for the future will lead to success. However, many medical groups understand perfectly well the descending spiral toward mediocrity and failure that their current path is taking them.

The vision for reinventing health care delivery outlined in this chapter should serve as a starting point for discussion and discourse within medical groups. By applying this vision against the current reality of care delivery offered by any medical group, challenging discussions will occur. Managers are encouraged to cultivate this discourse as a means to continually refine the essence of their group or clinic and to establish a beacon for guiding operations.

REFERENCES

Beck, M. & Salholz, E. (1993, April 5). Doctors under the knife. *Newsweek, 121*(14), 28–33.

Blumenthal, D. (1996, Summer). Effects of market reforms on doctors and their patients. *Health Affairs, 15*(2): 170–84.

Capitmann, J. A., Haskins, B., & Bernstein, J. (1986). Case management approaches in coordinated, community-oriented, long-term care demonstrations. *The Gerontologist, 26*, 398–404.

Crane, M. (1994). The malpractice dragon wasn't dead—just asleep. *Medical Economics, 71*(4), 52–59.

Davidson, S. M., McCollom, M., & Heineke, J. (1996). *The physician manager alliance: Building the health care organization.* San Francisco: Jossey-Bass.

Dolinsky, A. L. (1997). Elderly patients' satisfaction with the outcome of their health care complaints. *Health Care Management Review, 22*(2), 33–40.

Donabedian, A. (1980). *Explorations in quality assessment and monitoring: The definition of quality on approaches to its assessment* (Vol. 1). Ann Arbor, MI: Health Administration Press.

Eastaugh, S. R. (1986, November/December). Hospital quality scorecards, patient severity and the emerging value shopper. *Hospitals and Health Services Administration*, 85–102.

Ford, R. C., Bach, S. A., & Fottler, M. D. (1997). Methods of measuring patient satisfaction in health care organization. *Health Care Management Review, 22*(2), 74–89.

Fottler, M. D., Johnson, R. A., McGlown, K. J., & Ford, E. W. (1999). Attitudes of organized labor officials toward health care issues: An exploratory survey of Alabama labor officials. *Health Care Management Review, 24*(2), 71–82.

Freund, D. A., Ehrenhaft, P. M., & Hackbarth, M. (1984). *Medicaid reform: Four studies of case management.* Washington, DC: American Enterprise Institute.

Goes, J. B., & Zhan, C. (1995). The effects of hospital-physician integration strategies on hospital financial performance. *Health Services Research, 30,* 507–530.

Herzlinger, R. (1997). *Market driven health care.* Reading, MA: Addison-Wesley Publishing Company.

Hickson, G. B., Clayton, E. W., Githens, P. B., & Sloan, F. A. (1992). Factors that prompted families to file medical malpractice claims following perinatal injuries. *Journal of the American Medical Association, 217,* 1359–1363.

Hoy, E., Curtis, R., & Rice, T. (1991, Winter). Change and growth in managed care. *Health Affairs, 10,* 18–35.

Hughes, T. E., & Larson, L. N. (1991). Patient involvement in health care: A procedural justice viewpoint. *Medical Care, 29,* 297–303.

John, J. (1992). Patient satisfaction: The impact of past experience. *Journal of Health Care Marketing, 12*(3), 56–64.

Jun, M., Peterson, R. T., & Zsidisin, G. A. (1998). The identification and measurement of quality dimensions in health care: Focus group interview results. *Health Care Management Review, 23*(4), 81–96.

Kaldenberg, D. O., & Becker, B. W. (1999). Evaluations of care by ambulatory surgery patients. *Health Care Management Review, 24*(3), 73–81.

Krawlewski, J., Wingert, T., & Barbouche, M. H. (1996). Assessing the culture of medical group practices. *Medical Care, 34*(5), 377–388.

Lagoe, R. J., & Aspling, D. L. (1996). Enlisting physician support for practice guidelines in hospitals. *Health Care Management Review, 21*(4), 61–67.

Liedtka, J., & Whitten, E. L. (1997). Building better patient care services. *Health Care Management Review, 22*(3), 16–24.

Liedtka, J. M., & Whitten, E. (1998, March/April). Enhancing care delivery through cross-disciplinary collaboration: A case study. *Journal of Healthcare Management, 43*(2), 185–205.

Lowes, R. L. (1995, March 27). Are you expected to see too many patients? *Medical Economics,* 52–59.

Lowes, R. (1996, December 23). How a group's personality affects its members. *Medical Economics,* 35–47.

Lowes, R. L. (1998, April 13). Making midlevel providers click with your group. *Medical Economics,* 123–132.

Magnus, S. A. (1999). Physicians' financial incentives in five dimensions. *Health Care Management Review, 24*(1), 57–72.

Mechanic, D., & Schlesinger, M. (1996, June 5). The impact of managed care on patients' trust in medical care and their physicians. *JAMA, 275*(21): 1693–7.

Meighan, S. S. (1995). Where have all the primary care physicians gone? *Health Care Management Review, 20*(3), 64–67.

Pontes, M. C., & Pontes, N. M. H. (1997). Consumers' inferences about physician ability and accountability. *Health Care Management Review, 22*(2), 7–20.

Proenca, E. J. (1999). Employee reactions to managed care. *Health Care Management Review, 24*(2), 57–70.

Schneller, E. S. (1997). Accountability for health care. *Health Care Management Review, 22*(1), 38–57.

Shortell, S. M., Gillies, R., Anderson, D., Erickson, K., & Mitchell, J. (1996). *Remaking health care in America: Building organized delivery systems.* San Francisco: Jossey Bass.

Sonnad, S. S. (1998). Organizational tactics for the successful assimilation of medical practice guidelines. *Health Care Management Review, 23*(31), 30–37.

Succi, M. J., & Alexander, J. A. (1999). Physician involvement in management and governance. *Health Care Management Review, 24*(1), 33–44.

Trey, B. (1996). Managing interdependence on the unit. *Health Care Management Review, 21*(3), 72–82.

Unland, J. J. (1995, Winter). The evolution of physician-directed managed care. *Journal of Health Care Finance, 22*(2), 42–56.

U.S. healthcare rated poorly. (1992). *Marketing News, 26*(23), 1.

Yasin, M. M., Czuchry, A. J., Jennings, D. L., & York, C. (1999). Managing the quality effort in a health care setting. *Health Care Management Review, 24*(1), 45–56.

Young, G. J., Charns, M. P., Daley, J., Forbes, M. B., Henderson, W., & Khuri, S. (1997). Best practices for managing surgical services: The role of coordination. *Health Care Management Review, 22*(4), 72–81.

Chapter 3

A Physician-Based System of Care

Executive Summary

Most patients fondly remember a nostalgic relationship with their physician. They trusted the individual to provide the best care and to help them out of their illness. A physician was respected and knew each patient at a deeply personal level. This romantic view of physicians began to disappear due to the intersection of three dominant forces—new medical knowledge, payment policies and emphasis on quality of care. The rise of managed care has shaken to the very foundation the role of physicians in care delivery and the hallowed doctor-patient relationship.

To deliver the right care at the right time with kindness and caring at effective cost, physicians must be at the center of the care delivery model. The issue confronting medical groups is how to best construct practice arrangements to uplift the professional primacy of physicians while at the same time achieving operationally efficient care that is low-cost and high-quality.

To construct such systems and care delivery models, it is essential that the factors influencing physician decisions and the trends among these factors be thoroughly understood. This chapter reviews the explosion of scientific knowledge and how this explosion affects the options for structuring care between physicians and mid-level practitioners. Payment patterns are also examined in order to understand the impact on traditional care delivery processes and the need to create innovative thinking in the reconfiguration of care. Finally, insights are offered on how technology enables us to rethink the typical ways of serving patients.

Medical groups, their managers and physicians can aspire to and achieve more effective delivery systems by recognizing and attending to the pressures affecting medical care. However, a true shift in the paradigm of care delivery necessitates a willingness on the part of all parties to collaborate in defining a new model. As has been amply demonstrated, most managed care delivery systems have only touched upon the symptoms of the problems. Fresh thinking, especially regarding the role of an incorporation of physicians in problem solving, will be needed within medical groups in order to address present and future constraints.

THE CENTRALITY OF PHYSICIANS

Health care reform, whether in a medical group or for the system as a whole, will not work unless the restructuring is configured around physicians (Johnson, 1995). When all is said and done about changing health policies to encourage cost control, it is still the physician who performs the diagnosis and treatment for serious illnesses. Others in extended roles, such as nurse practitioners or physician assistants, can improve the productivity of physicians by completing fundamental diagnostic and primary care procedures. Patients who are not healthy want to receive care from someone who can alleviate their condition. They are not interested in the nuances of managed care. They do not want to hear excuses about why it will take several weeks to be seen before a diagnosis can be made or before treatment can begin. All they want is to become well.

A physician-based health care system implies that effective solutions to existing crises will be created with physicians at the center of resolutions (Colby, 1997). There still remains sufficient latitude to devise a functional care delivery system in which physicians provide leadership. A reinvented health system implies that past traditions of lofty salaries will be honored only if physician productivity is sufficient to merit high incomes. It suggests that the care delivery process will recognize and support the critical role of physicians in diagnosing and treating patients. However, it does not imply that physicians will perform all of the care delivery.

A physician-based health care system is centered around making better use of physicians and those ancillary providers who support them. The system of care will be structured to ensure that physicians focus on delivering quality care, that they treat a sufficient number of patients to achieve low-cost and high-quality care, and that patients will be the beneficiaries of an effective care delivery process (Goldfield, 1994).

THE EVOLUTION OF PHYSICIANS AND PHYSICIAN PRACTICES

The concept of how physicians can contribute to a highly functioning health system is complex. Yet, the role of physicians is crucial in understanding how to resolve the health care crisis by finding workable solutions that uplift providers, patients and payees alike. To begin this discussion, it is necessary to analyze who was drawn to medical care when a system did not exist, when physicians practiced in a cottage industry wherein the solo practitioner was paramount (Starr, 1982). Who were these individuals and what were their personalities, emotions and behaviors? Understanding these issues is important because those entering the medical profession today are attracted by many of these past expectations. Moreover, patients share many of these perceptions and expectations. Patients become upset when these promises are not fulfilled. When in the hospital, many patients still expect a kind and healing nurse to monitor their progress and are upset when a beeping machine replaces the nurse. They still expect that doctors will uphold their right to dignified and compassionate care. These perceptions and expectations must be addressed in a reinvented care delivery system.

Medical care has devolved into a dysfunctional system because of a number of forces. This demise has been haphazard and has not, by any means, resulted in a coherent effective system. Part of the dysfunctionality of health care delivery relates to the restraints placed on change because we are dealing with professionals and the ingrained expectations of both providers and patients. As suggested in Sidebar 3.1, physicians are now asked to perform in a cost-effective manner in order to emulate a business concerned with financial results (Woolhandler & Himmelstein, 1995). The strains on the improvised system are overwhelming. The question is whether or not providers will help transform the informal, haphazard, pseudo system into a fully integrated, comprehensive system.

An attempt should be made to understand: (1) Past expectations; (2) that which has changed, and (3) how these changes affect us now. By understanding these facts and relationships, we can retain everything of value and develop a new, effective system of health care that delivers high-quality care and yet is more cost effective. To do this, it is necessary to consider the character, emotions and behavior of physicians. Why do people choose a career in medicine? What do they hope to accomplish? What do they expect to receive in return for entering the medical profession? What strengths and weaknesses do they bring to the table that will impact the effort to develop a true system? All of these factors have an impact on doctors' desires and ability to change and their ability to work together as a group to implement the necessary changes. Historic professional idealism may tend to inhibit and make an effective transition more difficult. A physician-based system

SIDEBAR 3.1

Excessive Emphasis on Financial Goals: A Prescription for Balance

Has the health care system pendulum swung too far in favor of financial objectives to the exclusion of more traditional patient care goals? Woolhandler and Himmelstein argue that things have simply gotten out of hand in the health care system. They postulate a delivery system gone crazy and characterized by:

- Unemployed doctors seeking jobs;
- Those who are employed burdened with excessive patient loads;
- Referral avoidance;
- Practice guidelines that limit visits to seven minutes;
- Generous salaries contingent on corporate profits; and
- Millions of uninsured patients excluded from care.

Woolhandler and Himmelstein argue that managed care can evolve into patient care that is far superior to that which presently exists in society.

What changes are needed to de-emphasize the bottom line in patient care? Their suggestions reflect the sentiments of many physicians that existing physician resources can be put to better use:

- Trade off high physician salaries for more time spent with patients (that is, lower salaries in exchange for meaningful patient-physician visits);
- Use unemployed gastroenterologists to perform patient screening;
- Use jobless psychiatrists to address substance abuse and teenage suicide;
- Use idle ophthalmologists to remove cataracts; and
- Hire surgeons instead of surgical interns.

In short, Woolhandler and Himmelstein vent the frustration of many physicians who watch as managed care bureaucrats enforce policies that generate fiscal largesse while undermining every other dimension of desired health care—quality, accessibility and kindness.

Source: Adapted from S. Woolhandler & D. U. Himmelstein. (1995, Fall). The physician workforce delusion. *Health Affairs,* 279.

of care will address the traditions and assumptions and, in so doing, establish a solid foundation for enhanced care delivery that meets the expectations of patients, physicians and payors.

Overview of Physician Practice Changes

When physicians entered medicine 50 years ago, they could safely make a number of assumptions, as shown in Table 3.1. Medicine offered a long training period, but physicians could be independent once it was over. Physicians could become entrepreneurs and start their own businesses with a virtual guarantee of success. With few exceptions, they could begin their practice anywhere in the country and be assured of an income that was in the top 10 percent of all incomes in the nation. The practice (that is, the job) was secure and could not be taken away. Medicine was a generalist profession that encouraged broad thinking. Ideally, those who entered medicine were individuals who wanted to help others, and who would reap enormous emotional rewards.

Fifty years ago the goal of medicine was to provide the best care. Because all patients were different, medicine was realistically an art and a profession, so the definition of the best care was almost personal and unique. Other than long hours and limited freedom, there were few disadvantages to the practice of medicine. Moreover, if one were not entrepreneurial, there were jobs in the profession that were academic and others that involved salaried practice. In summary, for many people the medical profession provided an almost idyllic way of life involving creativity while rewarding physicians emotionally and making them financially secure and independent.

These factors are at the crux of the dilemma for most doctors today. There have been radical changes that physicians do not like (Deckard, 1995). Physicians are confused about the causes of their problem. They are doing their utmost to turn the clock back. Some wonder if it is their fault. Why has everything turned against them? What should they do? Consider what has happened or is about to happen with respect to the factors that made the medical profession so unique and wonderful as shown in Table 3.1.

Today there is still a long (or even longer) training period and mentoring process, but at the end physicians are not (and probably will never be) independent (Walsh & Borkowski, 1999). With few exceptions (for example, in very undesirable locations), the doctor

TABLE 3.1   Comparison of Changing Assumptions for Physician Practice

Assumptions for Physicians Entering Practice 50 Years Ago	Comparative Assumptions for Physicians Entering Practice Today
• Despite a long training period, physicians became independent clinicians once their training was complete.	• There are longer training periods, and in the end, physicians are not independent clinicians.
• Physician practices were entrepreneurial efforts with a virtual guarantee of success.	• With few exceptions, physicians cannot become entrepreneurs with guaranteed success.
• Physician practices could be initiated anywhere and generated high income with job security.	• Practices are not secure and high income is at risk.
• Medical practice was general in orientation.	• Medicine has become specialized even in primary practice.
• Medicine was altruistic, and physicians could gain enormous emotional rewards.	• Professional rewards have been constrained by cost and malpractice considerations.
• Other than long hours, there were few inherent disadvantages to medical practice.	• Long hours have been coupled with less freedom, which reduces the attractiveness of medical practice.
• The goal of practice was to provide the best care.	• The goal of providing the best care has been constrained by cost and malpractice considerations.
• Academic and salaried jobs were available to physicians who chose not to practice clinically.	• Most medical jobs in the future will be salaried.
• The medical profession provided an enormously rewarding personal life.	• The medical profession provides an emotionally challenging life.

cannot be entrepreneurial and start a practice with any chance of success. What happens to physicians' incomes is still an open question, but evidence is accumulating that income levels will decrease and drop from the top scale of national incomes. Jobs are not secure, and even those physicians who have developed a successful practice can lose it as a result of competitive and reimbursement pressures. After finishing medical school, doctors may be forced to go into areas of practice that they do not prefer.

There are still rewards in medicine today, but they are much more limited. As a result of cost and malpractice, there may be significant disincentives in both emotional and financial areas (Pontes & Pontes, 1997). The doctor may have a long-standing emotional relationship with a patient. Nonetheless, the patient may seek another provider because of lower cost. Physicians are discovering that patients are more likely to sue for malpractice because they were not satisfied with the results of the care they received. The goal is still to provide the best care, but several new aspects have entered the picture. First, the goal is the best care for the least cost (yet we do not know how to reach the goal or even the best approach to take). Second, malpractice is a coercive force that is pushing physicians to pursue the best standard of care regardless of the difference in patients. There is danger in being different and treating patients in a unique manner. Third, a significant part of the art of medicine is in diagnosis. However, diagnosis is increasingly made by tests rather than by physicians, so medicine is becoming a technology rather than an art. These three aspects of medical practice reinforce each other and have altered the fundamental art of medicine.

Today, the long hours and lack of freedom have improved as physicians work together. However, it is possible that the only way physicians can still develop a reasonable small practice is to locate in an undesirable area where they will have to work long hours with little freedom. At the very least, given the many factors threatening small practice survival, physicians will incur greater risk in maintaining the freedom and autonomy of their practices, as suggested in Sidebar 3.2 (Walker, 1997). Many of the medical jobs in the future will be salaried. It will be a buyers' market, so the remunerative and working conditions will not be like the ideal envisioned by aspiring medical students. It is possible that when all the turmoil in the health care delivery system is over and there is stability, the medical profession may again be emotionally and financially rewarding. This possibility is only one of several directions medical practice might take; no longer is a rosy future guaranteed.

The manner in which the changes finally galvanize will be based in large measure on how health care providers respond to the pressures. Will they resist the pressure to change, or will they accept the pressure and try to work out a result that provides the right care at the

SIDEBAR 3.2

Balancing the Benefits and Risks of Small Practices

If, as it has been estimated, only 15 percent of the senior market will be penetrated by large HMOs, then a tremendous opportunity exists for small practices and solo practitioners to serve Medicare beneficiaries. The small practice has many desirable attributes for serving this population, including the ability to:

- Establish a supportive relationship with patients who possess chronic diseases;
- Track patient health status and health maintenance activities;
- Create a system for tracking referrals;
- Compare the practice's patient panel with other patient populations in order to analyze utilization;
- Deliver preventive care;
- Ensure high patient satisfaction through service orientation;
- Provide convenient access and reliable coverage; and
- Track patient compliance.

In essence, the small practice can be better positioned to deliver the care that many seniors remember from years past.

The most serious challenge to small practices and managed care is the potential tendency to assume too much risk. One, or even a few, very sick patients could overwhelm the small practice. Consequently, some experts recommend that small groups join together in strategic alliances such as independent practice associations.

Source: L. M. Walker. (1997, April 7). What it takes for small practices to succeed. *Medical Economics, 99,* (104), 113–116.

right time with kindness at the lowest cost? Those care delivery goals (that is, performing the right care, time, kindness, cost) represent the essence of the field of health and medicine. Preventing what morbidity can be prevented, caring for the morbidity that cannot be prevented and relieving suffering represent the essence of medical practice. Despite the structural changes in medical practice, these common denominators of care will remain.

The response of physicians to these changes mimics the behavior that is expected when a person or group feels threatened and insecure. Basically, physicians are trying to prevent change at any cost. They are fighting to return to the past, to maintain their professional autonomy and to ensure their economic well-being. In the long run, these strategies will prove to be ineffective. Instead of fighting change, physicians need to embrace the opportunity to lead the reinvention of medical practice.

THE IMPACT OF NEW KNOWLEDGE ON PHYSICIAN SERVICES

One of the most significant, misunderstood and professionally non-managed problems in medicine is excessive knowledge. In many respects, this is probably the most ignored problem in the medical field today that has serious ramifications for sustaining a physician-based system of care. The medical system has grown enormously in parallel with scientific developments, resulting in a knowledge explosion that often overwhelms clinicians. This problem is exacerbated because many physicians maintain a set of beliefs that they feel should never be changed. In fact, the explosion in knowledge has made it imperative that some of medicine's sacred beliefs must be modified if physicians and other providers are to provide good care to people. However, instead of adapting to change and positively confronting the knowledge problem, the medical field has held on to sacred beliefs while simultaneously arguing that things are constantly getting better. Nonetheless, a study of generalists and specialists in Kansas City suggests that things are not getting better as far as the integration of new knowledge into medical practice (see Sidebar 3.3).

Knowledge Explosion in Medicine

In medicine, an explosion in new knowledge suggests taking a critical look at the way care is delivered. Nonetheless, such critical analysis has been slow to materialize because of the inertia surrounding physician practices. Historically, it was not beyond the capacity of a doctor

SIDEBAR 3.3

The Integration of New Medical Knowledge in General and Specialty Care

The rapid growth in medical knowledge is both a blessing and a curse. With new scientific discoveries come opportunities to improve diagnosis and treatment regimens. The ability to cure disease is the ultimate benefit from the explosion in scientific knowledge. However, there is a distinct problem in translating the science into practice. How can busy generalists and specialists keep apprised of the developments in their respective fields while also maintaining viable practices? This is a significant question considering the trend toward larger patient panels among managed care plans and the not-so-subtle pressures for increased productivity by providers. Where will physicians find the time to keep abreast of key developments and breakthroughs? How can they efficiently access information pertinent to their caseload or to specific patients? These are highly significant questions in view of the explosion of medical science.

Hunt and Newman surveyed physician access to medical knowledge among 691 family practitioners and specialists in Kansas City. Their findings are alarming because they imply that generalists not only have limited time to access information, but they also lack channels to routinely acquire information. First, the physicians report they have less time available than they did five years ago to read medical journals:

	Percentage Indicating		
	Less Time Available	*Same Time Available*	*More Time Available*
Generalists	80.2	12.0	7.3
Specialists	73.6	17.1	9.3

Clearly, if physicians do not read their journals they will be less cognizant of recent developments that could influence patient care.

Next, Hunt and Newman examined access to and use of medical information retrieval systems such as Medline or CD-ROM libraries. Generalists were less likely than specialists to have access to such systems. Those with access tended to lease their access. More discouraging

continued

was the limited use of information retrieval systems by both generalists and specialists:

		Percent Indicating		
	Never Use	**Use Less Than Once per Month**	**Use at Least Once per Month**	**Use at Least Once per Week**
Generalists	44	45	9	2
Specialists	10	46	30	13

In conclusion, physicians may not be able to remain current with medical knowledge advances. There is adequate technology available to assist physicians in learning about medical science developments; but it appears that time constrains the ability, or motivation, of physicians to access new medical knowledge.

Source: Adapted from R .E. Hunt & R. G. Newman. (1997). Medical knowledge overload: A disturbing trend for physicians. *Health Care Management Review, 22*(1), 70–75.

to possess all scientific knowledge for a specific illness. For the most part any single doctor could remain competent in all areas of medical care because the knowledge (scientific) base was relatively limited.

Beginning 60 years ago, specialization increased rapidly for several reasons. First, different doctors had different interests and liked to perform certain procedures more than others. Second, specialization evolved from skills as well as interests. Some physicians were more skillful at surgical operations and gravitated toward general surgery or obstetrics and gynecology. Others were more analytical and became drawn toward internal medicine or pediatrics. In specialty practice, physicians could know more about a narrow section of medical care compared to general practice. Third, as knowledge increased and skill application became more important, specialization expanded. Clear variations in the skills were observed among physicians. The increase in knowledge made these variations more apparent. These factors stimulated the wane of general physicians because, with the increase in new knowledge, one person could not be as skillful in all facets as someone who focused on one aspect of medical care.

As knowledge increased, specialization increased within specialties. Subspecialization arose because of knowledge, interest and skills. As knowledge increased, physicians focused on becoming experts in a narrower field. Actual care for any specific malady appeared to be better. However, a new problem developed. Total care of the entire person was lost in the rise of specialization. As specialties developed, general practice waned. In general, specialists had higher status, more prestige and made more money. Increasingly, hospitals excluded general practitioners from caring for inpatients.

As the medical system grew, no solid method was created for cultivating and maintaining relationships among specialists. Patients could drop through the cracks between specialists and sometimes did so with disastrous results. Moreover, as science came into medical care, kindness and care for the patient decreased. Consequently, there was no one to provide security and understanding for patients.

In large part due to these trends, a resurgence occurred within family practice. Physicians were subsequently specifically trained for this new specialty. A logical offshoot was the recognition that patients should have a primary physician. This primary caregiver would be someone patients knew on an ongoing basis and who would correlate care. The primary provider also served as a source of kindness or compassion that had been lost in medicine. The primary caregiver would enable patients to see appropriate specialists at the right time. Primary providers tended to correct that which had been lost when patients went directly to specialists, but reliance on primary providers did not solve the underlying knowledge problem.

New Knowledge and a Physician-Based System of Care

With respect to medical knowledge, there is now too much for any one person to know (Hunt & Newman, 1997). Philosophically, there are two approaches for addressing this problem. One person with general knowledge can care for the patient and then refer him or her to a specialist while still coordinating the care. Alternatively, in some manner the patient is sent to the appropriate specialists immediately and the nonphysician sender coordinates the care. In the first situation, the provider has relationship, triage and care functions whereas in the second situation, the provider, who typically is not a physician, has only relationship and triage functions. Which model functions best is really a philosophical question. However, the target for a functional health delivery system should be the system that results in the best care, gives the patient the most confidence and is the least expensive.

There are certain different prerequisites with either approach. The first, or traditional, system must be based on a rewarding relationship between patient and care provider. The provider must have knowledge and be able to triage the patient through a complex system. The provider must be a doctor with general knowledge in the area of care (that is, internist, family physician or pediatrician) because all possible care will be provided by this person. Finally, clinicians must be able to determine when they need help and should consult or refer the patient to specialists. There should be no barriers to referral if the patient is to receive the best care. Unfortunately, in many current managed care systems, such barriers to referral are all too prevalent.

Intellectually and emotionally, the traditional approach to care delivery is quite a task for one physician. Nonetheless, without effective doctor-patient relationships, the care delivery process begins to break down. In addition to being able to maintain effective, long-term relations with patients, providers must also triage effectively. This can be done personally or delegated with specific direction, but triage is time consuming. On top of these constraints, the provision of care may be highly difficult. In the past, a good patient-physician relationship was automatic and providing care was all the doctor had to do. There was just one thing to think about—treatment. Now with costs as a dominant consideration, care is more complicated and becomes interrelated with triage. The doctor must know when referral is desirable. That decision is subject to review and must correlate with the judgment of the specialist. Critical analysis suggests that in the traditional system, there are too many different agendas for one person to be concerned with if the best care is to result. The system is too complicated and should be broken down into component parts.

In the second system, there are still the same basic functions of patient relationship, triage and care, yet they are separated. The basis of this system is that the provider fulfilling the patient relationship and performing triage does not have to be a doctor. In this second system, patients develop a rewarding relationship with a provider. This goal is easily accomplished if the provider is knowledgeable (for example, nurse practitioner), but not necessarily a physician (Keeprews, 1995). The provider must have sufficient intelligence and training to effectively undertake the triage function. The triage person essentially becomes the patient's advocate in assisting him or her into and through the complicated system. The triage provider must have sufficient authority to get the patient in contact with a physician at any time (for example, authority to make emergency appointments with the appropriate physician). In many cases, the necessary physician will be determined based on the patient's complaints. When it is not, the triage person discusses the patient's problems with a physician who provides oversight and ensures that the correct contact is made. A critical distinguishing aspect of the second system is that patients must be satisfied with the outcome of care delivery. There should be no instances in which the patient believes a doctor visit is necessary, and after receiving care from a nonphysician provider, still believes that seeing a physician is imperative.

The second system allows triage providers to refer patients to specialists early (as appropriate) and, thus, focuses more expertise on their problem initially. Because there is too much knowledge in the medical field for anyone to master, this approach provides a definite advantage. It also cultivates a rewarding relationship and provides the patient with an expert who can help negotiate a complicated network. This person who triages the patient through the system will ensure that the patient is not lost. Basically, it is a plan to solve the problems of a good relationship while incorporating specialization.

A physician-based system of care should build constructively on the developments in new knowledge and technology surfacing from the scientific community. In the final analysis, the issue is really not a choice of whether physicians or mid-level providers (with strong reporting relationships to physicians) lay hands on patients. **The critical question is whether the health delivery system receives leadership from physicians in order to capitalize on new knowledge, technological breakthroughs and innovative methods of configuring mid-level providers under physician supervision.**

Equally effective and ineffective physician-centered delivery models are found throughout the health care delivery system. Care delivery by physicians is not a panacea. However, given the continuing research that leads to new medical knowledge and technology that must be integrated into clinical care, physicians certainly are best positioned for leadership. In a reinvented health care system, physicians would be comfortable with their ability to delegate routine care delivery to mid-level providers (while maintaining appropriate checks and balances). They would have more time to focus on new knowledge and technology that would increase their productivity and quality of care while assisting others and the care delivery system to do likewise.

THE IMPACT OF PAYMENT ON PHYSICIAN SERVICES

To this point, the centrality of physicians in reinvented health delivery systems has been considered from several perspectives: the evolution of physician practice, why private practices worked well in the past, why physicians have become alienated with the present system and how medical practice has been affected by the influx of new scientific knowledge. Payment for physician services differs from many of these other factors in one respect—methods of payment evolved over a much shorter period of time. Reimbursement for physician services was a dramatic change instituted by third parties including the government and private insurers. Insurance coverage via fee-for-service methods seemed to be a step in the right direction because it relieved patients from onerous financial burdens while ensuring fiscal remuneration for physicians. Evidence is accumulating, however, that it may have been a step in the wrong direction. The cost of medical care is a significant issue that may be destroying our health care system. It is the single factor that many feel will destroy the medical system. The dysfunctional consequences of fee-for-service are depicted in Figure 3.1.

Although fee-for-service payment has contributed to the health care cost crisis, reimbursement could also become the most important factor in saving the health care system. Fee-for-service payments have stimulated the debate about the entire health care system (Heshmat, 1997). If, as a nation, we have the courage to do what is possible, we could end up with a far more efficient system that delivers high quality of care. There is hope and certainty of success, but the path to success is very narrow. However, there is truly opportunity in crisis. To capitalize on this opportunity, it is important to go back in time to determine how fee-for-service began to drive up the cost of care, and how costs can now be moderated without impairing the health care that individuals receive.

The inability of physicians to leave behind the perquisites of a fee-for-service milieu created a vacuum that, in turn, was filled by managed care. The managed care concept seemed to provide some

<table>
<tr><td>Two-tiered system</td><td>*Wealthy Patients Receive Care from Private Physicians*</td><td>*Patients Who Have Financial Constraints Receive Care from Hospital Clinics*</td></tr>
</table>

Two-
tiered
system

Wealthy Patients Receive Care from Private Physicians

Patients Who Have Financial Constraints Receive Care from Hospital Clinics

- There is no uniformity in fees charged by physicians.
- Patients are assigned to private hospital rooms with many amenities.

- Physicians offer their services at low or no cost.
- Prominent physicians restrict their practices to private patients.
- Clinic patients are assigned to hospital wards without amenities.

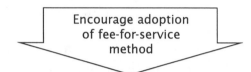

Encourage adoption
of fee-for-service
method

Specific services are worth specific fees regardless
of who the patient is or the provider.
Fees are initially based on time invested and complexity of procedure.

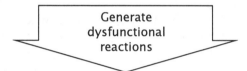

Generate
dysfunctional
reactions

- Range of fees is narrowed, but prominent physicians receive higher fees for services.
- Hospital clinics close as physicians are less able to afford free care.
- Amenities of hospital care (nursing care, food, privacy) become rights for all patients.
- Despite little differentiation in quality of care, services are bundled to generate significant charge differences.
- Medical care and physician services are expanded to cover every possible contingency.
- Specialized tasks require highly specialized fees.
- Providers equate payment with cost.

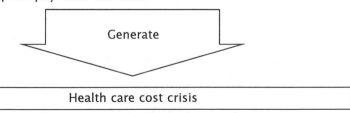

Generate

Health care cost crisis

Figure 3.1   Fee-For-Service Payments and the Health
Care Cost Crisis

hope because HMOs were concerned with costs, which in turn placed restraints upon how doctors (and hospitals) practiced medicine. Care was managed and there was a ceiling on what could be spent. The HMO was at risk for the cost of care. However, physicians have allowed the control of medical care to be assumed by managed care plans and were dramatically affected by HMOs, as discussed in Sidebar 3.4.

Cost reduction is occurring in two ways. HMOs have a global, yearly fee so, in a sense, they have instituted a fee ceiling on physician income. Buyers of health care services (for example, employees) are negotiating to reduce this fee and capitate the HMOs at a reduced rate. This brings business-type price negotiation into health care for the first time. Tough contract negotiations may be good from a cost reduction point of view, but if the HMO does not know how to reduce the cost of the care, it may not be good for physicians or patients. The consequence is that physicians must modify their practice patterns to meet the demands of the insurers.

The other way that HMOs are coping with cost reduction is to have patients pay a greater share of the cost of the care. This approach jeopardizes the management of care and threatens to increase health costs over the long run. From the beginning, HMOs had patient copayments for some types of care in order to discourage patients from overusing the system. Copayments for office visits might be only a few dollars. Copayments for emergency department use or elective operations might be $50 or $100. HMOs are now adding copayments for different services and increasing the amount of copayments that have been in effect.

Another method of reducing cost is a subtle form of rationing care. In most HMOs, patients have a primary physician who is a family physician or internist by training and is responsible for the family. This primary physician is a gatekeeper who must make all referrals to specialists. The primary physicians may have guidelines to meet as a gatekeeper with financial incentives to meet the guidelines. These guidelines may be set in relation to national benchmarks (that is, a specific number of cholecystectomies in the population, a cesarean section rate below 15 percent, etc.) and may have no relationship to the core of patients to which a particular primary physician is responsible for delivering care. The result is that someone with gallbladder symptoms might be encouraged to wait as long as possible before receiving an operation. Whether or not this is the best medical care is

SIDEBAR 3.4

The Physician Reaction to Managed Care

It is difficult to use research surveys to precisely capture the angst and hard feelings that physicians express about the managed care practice environment. Somehow, the numbers and percentages cannot quite reflect the resentment that many physicians feel concerning the changes before their profession. Nonetheless, there is a definite sense of alienation and anger among physicians who realize that the business of health care has come to dominate the practice of medicine. The *New England Journal of Medicine* often publishes letters and notes from physicians regarding the transitions in medicine. Following are excerpts from a letter by Dr. Philip R. Alper, an internist, who eloquently expresses in a tongue-in-cheek manner the positive aspects of managed care. Dr. Alper's cynical parody of the positive outcomes of managed care undoubtedly receives widespread emotional support from many colleagues.

"Learning to accentuate the positive in managed care."

Philip R. Alper

New England Journal of Medicine, February 13, 1997, 336(7), 508–509.

Managed care scares me, but with patients enrolled in health maintenance organizations (HMOs) now making up a quarter of my internal-medicine practice, I've found it essential to think positive thoughts. This often means discerning silver linings where others see only clouds.

Flexibility is essential. Once, I believed that only the physicians treating patients should define and take charge of their care. Managed care has successfully challenged this philosophy by showing that patients (and doctors) are more similar than they are different. Also, I have learned that an obsessive concentration on the doctor-patient relationship distracts me from attending to the needs of the unseen others for whom the carrier has assumed contractual responsibility.

Thus, we have the managed-care credo that in order to worry best about everyone in general, it's essential not to worry too much about anyone in particular. Just remember that nobody is special, and the rest comes naturally. My new concern about populations of patients rather than mere individuals has expanded my own horizons. I feel a greater kinship with the HMO experts who work hard

continued

to maintain this focus. Sometimes I marvel at my former narrow-mindedness.

To be sure, long-time patients and the people they referred to me, often with a middle-class perspective similar to my own, were comfortable to treat. As we aged together, I often knew what my patients were going to say even before they said it. Illnesses that I believed I could treat effectively seemed to become more common in my practice

Now, with HMO patients assigned to me on a rotating basis, I see the full spectrum of medical and social problems. And so do my old patients, who encounter all kinds of interesting new people in the waiting room. My new, less differentiated practice reminds me of my internship, I feel younger and more vigorous as a result.

In addition, I find it a challenge to see patients who never heard of me until they got my name out of a directory of providers. In the past, suspicion and hostility from patients were so rare that I hadn't developed any proficiency in dealing with them. (I was actually prone to consider these traits possible signs of paranoia.) Now I have reason to reconsider: What about the psychological effects of heavy exposure to the media's horror stories about managed care? Are the patients paranoid or just scared?

Getting suspicious patients to like me while still doing my job as a gatekeeper—which mainly means getting them not to want what they can't have—is a test of my professionalism. I like conjuring up the right words to allay their fears about the rationing of care and about undertreatment. The challenge has reinvigorated many a humdrum day. No chance of boredom or burnout for me!

Of course, there's also the issue of money. I believe managed care is the perfect antidote to greed in physicians. It takes a little getting used to, but I've found it much healthier just to forget about money. At first, it concerned me that the lower fees and fewer reimbursable services of managed care brought in much less income. Now I look on the bright side—come what may, I'll probably still have enough to pay the rent, my staff's salaries, and the telephone bills. Besides, people who resented physicians' high incomes in recent years will probably find me more socially acceptable this way.

Minimizing my concern about my own financial prospects also keeps me from getting too worked up over all the expensive ads that HMOs put on television, radio, and billboards and in the newspapers. I figure the companies probably know best how to deploy their resources, since their business is business and mine is only medicine. Of course, by keeping doctors busy and not overpaying them, they eliminate the temptation to overtreat patients for financial reasons.

The companies have become very good at this. I recently read in the *Wall Street Journal* that U.S. Healthcare pays its doctors 1.5 percent

continued

more per patient per month if they work 50 to 60 hours a week.[1] Imagine! Time and a half replaced by time and a 50th! Whatever works!

Learning to ignore money in the midst of an "only money talks" world builds character. Some doctors get discouraged by the pressure this creates, however. To them I say that it puts doctors on a par with everyone else. After all, pilots and engineers know what it's like to be in great demand one year and a glut on the market the next. Doctors should expect good times and bad times just like other people. Humility is also a great asset in caring for patients.

I will concede, however, that doctors' egos do need a boost from time to time. What better way than to take pride in being part of a greater cause than ours alone? The independent practice association to which I belong contracts with 13 HMOs. All of them boast in the papers and on television about the quality of the doctors in their plans and how much we all care about every patient in the plan. I figure that since I'm a part of all 13 teams, I must be a pretty darn good doctor, with access to an awful lot of patients. It makes me feel important.

Another ego boost has come from my promotion from a mere internist to a "primary care provider," the new way for us to be addressed. No longer just an internist, I'm now also a skilled psychiatrist, gynecologist, dermatologist, and even orthopedic surgeon. Whatever my doubts about my abilities, I forge ahead with confidence. The HMOs have taught me to believe I can do whatever they say I can.

In fact, the HMOs go out of their way to be helpful. Three different protocols telling me how to take care of patients with diabetes have come in the mail, and more are on the way. The HMOs' medical directors send bulletins explaining the right way to treat all kinds of other illnesses, including congestive heart failure. I like it when they tell us what drugs to prescribe, particularly when they include the dosages (a Blue Shield innovation). Checking the mail to see what new help has arrived is a highlight of every day.

I treasure such assistance because in the past, with medical students to teach and a practice to look after, I had far too many things to figure out and remember. Now I can lean back and relax a little. I receive advisories on almost everything. I'll admit that it gets a little confusing at times to figure out which patient is in which HMO so I know how to treat the disease according to the right advisory. Juggling 15 different drug formularies and 3 different sets of preventive-care guidelines (so far) is also a challenge. The bright side is that it's an excellent memory-enhancer.

Managed care works surprisingly hard to sharpen our memories. Those 13 HMOs that our group deals with sell 1200 different types of insurance contracts to our patients. When the patients call,

continued

remembering who's in what plan and with which contract (so I can determine what's allowed and what isn't) is a wonderful mental exercise, especially on nights and weekends. It's like an IQ test. And if a doctor gets lonely, the big piles of mail from HMOs are a comfort. It's a pity there just isn't time to do it all justice.

Even my office staff is sharing in the benefits of managed care. They used to be compulsive about keeping the office accounts. This is no longer necessary, since we no longer know how much we're going to be paid. The staff gets plenty of laughs from out-of-date insurance-eligibility lists. It sets them to playing detective. Our practice association explains that giving back money we thought we had earned is not a problem, because it is more than likely to be offset by other payments that we're not entitled to. "Everything evens out in the end," they say. I think this is a good way to look at it. The staff is so much more easygoing. Patients seem to be happier, too.

I don't want to seem like a complainer, but I do have one negative item to report. The other day I attended a conference on managed care. "We're far from the bottom of the market for physician reimbursement," one of the speakers said. To prove his point that there's plenty of room for an even greater downward earnings spiral, he added, "You don't see many doctors filing for bankruptcy or jumping off bridges yet."

This does sound a little mean to me, and I sure hope I'm not one of the ones he's talking about. But even if I am, with my new positive outlook, I know it's for a good cause.

"Next patient, nurse."

References

1. A special background report on trends in industry and finance. *Wall Street Journal*. August 1, 1996:A1.

questionable, but it is often more expensive if long-term rather than short-term results are concerned.

From a cost reduction point of view, the HMO concept with a specific fee is a step in the right direction. It certainly instills a greater incentive for cost control than that found in fee-for-service payments. HMOs present opportunities to standardize some aspects of care, to write protocols and to provide less complex and better care. The HMO concept has many similarities with the model that has been so successful in business; that is, the multispecialty functional team. Unfortunately, there are many forces that operate against HMOs in their efforts to utilize multispecialty functional teams. Most of these pressures can be linked to traditions centered around concepts of what is required to deliver the best care. These are traditions and beliefs that perpetuate the health care crisis.

As medical groups and physicians look to the future of health care, they should remember the past, particularly the former policy changes that have driven the health system to its current position. All too often, HMOs were touted as the final solution to the impending crisis. History sadly demonstrates that a single intervention cannot resolve all problems. Powerful interventions such as HMOs, managed care, prospective payment and similar strategies are only pieces in the final puzzle. It can be argued that the most indelible solutions will occur at the provider level. Medical groups and physicians occupy the positions from which fundamental change can evolve and from which the health care system can transcend to a new level. However, physicians must act in a concerted way to bring a financially viable health system that delivers quality care and in which physicians play a pivotal role in the structure, process and outcome of care.

THE IMPACT OF QUALITY AND TECHNOLOGICALLY ADVANCED CARE ON PHYSICIAN SERVICES

Medicine appears to be in the early stages of an industrial revolution. A number of forces are coming together to make this kind of change in medicine. If used effectively, technology can influence cost, who does what (that is, who provides care) and the level of productivity for physicians and other providers. Increased use of medical technology is a deterrent to malpractice. Medical technology tends to produce numbers or visual images that are often considered hard evidence. Whether right or wrong, technology gives the impression of hard evidence rather than someone's judgment that gives the impression of soft evidence. Moreover, new technology is embraced and desired by the public due to advertising by the manufacturers of the technology. All of these factors seem to be converging to support more medical technology and probably less human effort in the practice of medicine. Nonetheless, physicians often seem to ignore these trends. Much of primary care in the future may be delivered by technology. Physicians should prepare for this future by carefully defining how technology will be used to support physician-based care.

The Evolution of Medical Technology

New medical discoveries have become a distinguishing reality of health care (Prince, 1998). At first, doctors could do little but be kind, care for patients and relieve pain. Early medical discoveries were focused on finding causes of specific diseases, perfecting new operations and disseminating the new knowledge. Changes occurred in about 1920. Doctors began to acquire sufficient scientific knowledge so that they could really help patients and do more than be kind and relieve pain. In some ways, the decades from 1920 to 1960 were the age of the doctor. Many of the fundamental concepts about how medicine ought to be practiced arose from this period. The hallmark of this period was the sanctity of the doctor's judgment. There were many options for care. The doctor's job as an expert was to utilize the best judgment in choosing a correct option for services.

Then, about 1960, with increasing scientific discoveries, technology began to replace judgment. In some instances, doctors needed to use no judgment. The patient would describe symptoms and, from this description, the doctor could order some specific tests. The physician would confirm the diagnosis at a subsequent visit and, therefore, the necessary treatment. In essence, this was a simple progression from question to answer: symptoms → tests → test results → diagnosis → treatment → patient cured. Increasingly, algorithms were followed using specific tests. However, the heritage of medicine continues to honor the judgment of physicians as the hallmark of quality care.

The diagnosis and treatment of ectopic pregnancy is a good example of how one serious entity has been reduced to a minor problem with technology. Three technologies are involved: ultrasound, quantitative pregnancy tests and laparoscopy. Prior to the development of these technologies, ectopic (tubal) pregnancy was suspected when a woman had irregular bleeding and abdominal pain in early pregnancy. She could have bleeding with a threatened spontaneous abortion and cramping pain. Often the diagnosis was not clear, and the abdomen had to be opened at operation to see the distended tube and make the diagnosis. It was dangerous to wait because sometimes there was fatal bleeding when the tube ruptured with an ectopic pregnancy.

Now the condition is much easier to diagnose and treat. If suspected, ultrasound will show whether or not there is an intrauterine pregnancy. If so, it is very unlikely that the patient also has an ectopic pregnancy (probability of 1 in 40,000). Tubal pregnancy is not well visualized on ultrasound; so if the patient has no intrauterine pregnancy with a positive pregnancy test, it is probable that there is a pregnancy in the tubes. Quantitative pregnancy tests can then be completed every 24 to 48 hours. Some tubal pregnancies die and are resorbed, so the serial pregnancy tests go down in strength. If the tests rise, laparoscopy can be utilized to make a specific diagnosis and remove the tube. Technology has made possible accurate diagnosis and treatment without a major operation.

THE IMPERATIVE FOR A PHYSICIAN-BASED SYSTEM

The demise of the perfect physician and the perfect practice, usually a solo practice, has been brought about by many factors. Increased medical knowledge, fee-for-service payments and the emphasis on quality care and new technology represent important changes in medicine that significantly changed the landscape of the profession. Today, physicians and their patients are confronted by a corporate system of care based around large managed care plans (Bodenheimer & Sullivan, 1998). It appears that few, if any, providers are pleased with the situation that now controls their medical practices. While resourceful physicians continue to develop strategies allowing them to survive within the changing health care context, there is a growing set of constraints on any single practitioner (Bindman, Grumbach, Uranizan, Jaffe, & Osmond, 1998). The result is widespread dissension and dissatisfaction about the profession.

The most serious concern among physicians appears to be a sense of loss of control over the ability to practice as they deem appropriate. In a study of young physicians, Hadley and Mitchell concluded that managed care had a significant, adverse impact on physician satisfaction, as shown in Figure 3.2 (Hadley & Mitchell, 1997). Their findings suggest that physicians altered their clinical practice behaviors in response to HMO penetration and consequently lowered physician satisfaction with their efforts at care delivery. The results have been confirmed in other studies that document the limitations that HMOs place on clinical decisionmaking (National Opinion Research Center, 1995).

The startling finding from Hadley and Mitchell's study is that HMO penetration not only reduces physician satisfaction with

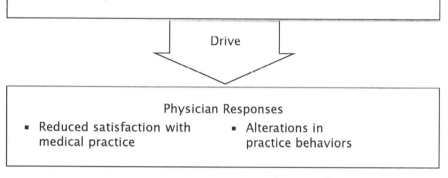

Doubling the HMO penetration has unusual practice effects:
- 4% fewer annual practice hours
- 14% fewer patients seen per week
- 20% greater likelihood of not being satisfied with one's practice
- Erosion of practice income

Drive

Physician Responses
- Reduced satisfaction with medical practice
- Alterations in practice behaviors

FIGURE 3.2   The Impact of Managed Care on Physicians

Source: Adapted from J. Hadley & J. Mitchell. (1997). Effects of HMO market penetration on physicians' work effort and satisfaction. *Health Affairs.*

medical practice, but it also alters practice behaviors. Physicians report that they work fewer hours per week and that they see fewer patients per week, ostensibly because they are dissatisfied with the type of practice environment created by HMOs. This milieu also carries a negative impact on practice income. The results of this study have two major limitations because the sample included only those physicians under the age of 45 years and because the data was cross-sectional. Nonetheless, the conclusions surfacing from the study mimic the results from other, broader national surveys.

The inevitable conclusion from the studies that examine the impact of managed care on physicians and patients is that undesired outcomes are surfacing (Blumenthal, 1996; Kuttner, 1998). Figure 3.3 presents this paradox as a drive toward substandard care. Managed care is producing clinical mediocrity because it places great constraints on how physicians practice medicine. Gatekeeping functions within HMOs strain physician-patient relationships because the primary physician must essentially tell patients that they cannot receive specialty care or they must enter specialty care after experiencing serious delays. Physicians are less able to create a treatment plan that

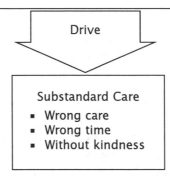

Physician Concerns about Organizational Constraints
- Gatekeeping strains physician-patient relationship by denial of access to specialty care.
- Utilization review interferes with the process of matching services to individual patient needs.
- Practice guidelines cannot take into account patient and physician preferences for care.
- Risk-sharing threatens medical practice in several ways:
  - Physicians may underserve patients in order to reduce costs;
  - Physicians (and managed care organizations) may avoid costly patients; and
  - Physicians do not have a sufficient actuarial risk spread (86% of primary care physicians do not have reinsurance or "stop-loss" protection).

Drive

Substandard Care
- Wrong care
- Wrong time
- Without kindness

FIGURE 3.3   Managed Care Producing Clinical Mediocrity

Sources: Adapted from D. Blumenthal. (1996). Effects of market reforms on doctors and their patients. *Health Affairs, 15*(2):170–89. R. Kuttner. (1998). Must good HMOs go bad? *New England Journal of Medicine, 338*(21): 1558–63.

matches specific, individual patient needs due to clinical practice guidelines established by managed care plans or due to utilization review processes that override the recommendations of physicians.

Managed care plans further constrain care delivery through guidelines that do not account for patient or physician preferences for care. To illustrate, a patient with a large renal calculus may wish to receive lithotripsy, a desire that is supported by the patient's primary care physician. However, if the calculus does not meet the minimum threshold for size, then the managed care plan will not approve the procedure. If that patient has numerous international travel plans, she or he may be traveling with a timebomb that is about to explode.

Finally, Figure 3.3 suggests that risk-sharing by physicians involved in managed care plans may adversely affect clinical practice. Patients stand to lose in several ways, including the inability to receive needed services (as physicians reduce care in order to reduce costs) and the inability to access some providers who suspect that the patients are too costly and thus, are a financial risk to them under a capitated arrangement (for example, patients with chronic illnesses). Physicians also stand to lose from risk-sharing if they do not have reinsurance stop-loss protection, which actually provides a "ceiling" for risk for those few expensive cases with catastrophic expenses. These consequences of managed care hardly promote the concept of the right care at the right time with kindness, although admittedly the low cost goal is achieved.

A PHYSICIAN-BASED MODEL OF CARE

Physicians can regain their control of medicine and the health care system, but it will require an entirely different mindset than that used to this point in response to managed care (Guptill Warren, Weitz, & Kulis, 1999). They will essentially have to move toward a new model of thinking about care delivery. Uwe Reinhardt argues that the most important decision facing physicians in this regard will be with whom they will affiliate for care delivery (*Medical Economics*, 1996). Reinhardt observes that most physicians inherently do not trust hospitals, or the incentives that drive hospitals. This distrust is certainly fueled by adverse physician relations with managed care organizations, as exemplified in Sidebar 3.5. Physicians are better served by affiliation in physician organizations that optimally represent their interests and philosophy of care delivery (Burns, 1996). However, affiliation is only the starting point. Physicians and physician leaders are challenged to provide an improved model of care delivery that achieves low cost while simultaneously producing the right care at the right time with kindness (Unland, 1995).

Why, when all indicators point to physician loss of control of medicine, is it imperative that physicians regain their preeminence in leadership? **In the final analysis, it is the physician who is the critical player—the one who blends the art and science of medicine; the**

SIDEBAR 3.5

The Fight for a Physician-Based Practice

Many physicians argue that managed care companies have rendered care delivery to the level of a financial question rather than an issue of quality. Managed care is accused of debasing physician-patient relations and substituting the bottomline as the criterion for measuring health care delivery success. The result is a palpable contention between physicians and medical management. Nowhere was this battle more evident that with the Thomas-Davis Medical Center in Tucson, Ariz. The following case study merely illustrates the contentious relations that have arisen between management and physicians; a contentiousness that must be resolved in order to benefit patients, physicians and the bottom line.

"When the fighting's over, will this practice still be standing?"

David Azevedo

Medical Economics, March 23, 1998, 166–167.

Among the plaques and artwork that hang in the lobby of FPA Medical Management's national headquarters in San Diego is a framed T-shirt that reads: "Today's Determination May Bring Tomorrow's Cure." Each of the capital letters is a different color, and together they form TDMC, the initials of Thomas-Davis Medical Centers, a Tucson-based multispecialty group.

FPA, a publicly traded management-services organization, purchased the group in late 1996. Since then, the MSO's executives have embarked on a determined effort to find a cure for the group's diseased finances. FPA officials say the group had been losing up to $2 million a month.

Some Thomas-Davis doctors believe that FPA, far from trying to save the patient, is trying to kill it—or at least cut off a few essential limbs. Indeed, entire departments have been shut down in favor of contracting with community doctors. And although no doctors were laid off, during the first 15 months of FPA's management, more than half the group's 219 doctors retired or simply quit.

Thomas-Davis made national news least year when its physicians joined the Tallahassee, Fla.-based Federation of Physicians and Dentists to collectively bargain with management.* The doctors had been reeling from changes—such as increasing physicians' workloads, while at the same time slashing salaries and reducing servic-

continued

es to patients—made since they sold the clinic and its prominent HMO, called Intergroup, in 1994 to Foundation Health, a large California-based HMO (now part of Foundation Health Systems). The sale brought each TDMC physician shareholder $3.3 million. In late 1996, Foundation sold the physician group to FPA.

Even though the National Labor Relations Board certified the union, FPA at first refused to bargain, arguing that the doctors are supervisors and therefore ineligible to unionize. Last September, a federal district court ordered the company to come to the table.

Negotiations have yet to produce a contract—hardly an unexpected development, in light of the fact that on crucial issues the two sides remain far apart. The doctors resent what they consider FPA's assumption that they're lazy and unproductive. They believe the MSO has been heavy-handed in its approach to the clinic and is more interested in bullying its management strategies into place than engaging in partnership with employees. And those strategies, the doctors claim, are purely profit-driven and threaten the integrity of practitioners and the health of patients.

FPA insists it's simply trying to reverse Thomas-Davis's dismal financial position by applying managed-care tactics that have worked in other markets. Quality isn't compromised, FPA officials say emphatically; if it were, HMOs wouldn't send patients.

FPA Chief Executive Officer Seth Flam, a family practitioner, summed up the company's stance in a recent letter to San Diego Physician magazine: "These physicians are reacting less as a result of some feeling of moral obligation to their patients, and more as a result of their unwillingness to adapt to nationwide changes."

Can management and the union co-exist? The answer may not come for a while. Given the depth of feeling on both sides, the cure— if there is one—will be found only after a long and painful course of treatment.

---

one who provides the treatment and the cure; and the one with whom patients establish a relationship. A physician-based system of care is part of the answer due to the excesses brought about by managed care. As Figure 3.4 suggests, both patients and employers—the purchasers of medical care—are alarmed about the one-sided focus on cost. In the future, greater attention will be given to the ability of managed care plans to produce high quality and low cost (Herzlinger, 1998). Physicians are the critical determinant of a managed care plan's performance on these two dimensions.

The managed care scorecard displays both positive and negative results. On the one hand, capitated care has lowered the rate of health

The Managed Care Scorecard

Positive Results from Managed Care:

- Lowered rate of health insurance premiums leading to leveled costs

Adverse Results from Managed Care:

- Lower patient satisfaction;
- Lower quality; and
- Less access.

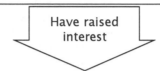

Have raised interest

Emphasis on Quality of Care

- Businesses will demand more than just low-cost care (they will seek value).
- Opportunities will emerge for medium-sized delivery systems that are small enough to create a culture of cost control and quality, yet large enough to accept risk.
- Quality will mean more than just applying clinical practice guidelines; teams and multiple treatment options will be necessary to achieve quality.

FIGURE 3.4

Source: How doctors can regain control of health care. *Medical Economics* (1996, May 13), 176–201.

insurance premium increases. In effect, this can be interpreted broadly as lowering costs. This gain is balanced against adverse results from managed care including lower patient (and provider) satisfaction, lower quality, and less access. In short, managed care has driven an obsession with costs and few of the other outcomes of health care delivery. Employers (who fund much of private health insurance) and patients are vitally interested in the quality of care as well as its cost. What good is low cost if a person does not improve?

In the future, more businesses will demand managed care plans to document their performance relative to quality indicators. Businesses will seek those plans that deliver value for the health care expenditure—a balance of both quality and cost. This implies opportunity for small- and medium-sized managed care plans that can create a culture of cost control and quality control yet are large enough to accept and thrive under risk (Kralewski et al., 1998). An emphasis on quality will also mean a robust setting for care delivery—a setting where physicians have latitude to treat patients in a variety of ways.

The prognosis for a physician-based system of care is very good. Physicians are the pivotal point for the reinvention of medical practice. **However, it is incumbent on medical professionals that they rise to the occasion to demonstrate leadership that is consistent with their central role.** This can be achieved by physicians (and physician leaders) working in concert with their medical groups. We believe that medical groups can transcend the pressures if physicians make intelligent choices about their practice settings and the configuration of medical practice processes and structures. Consequently, the implications for physicians and medical group presented in Table 3.2 are particularly poignant because they offer guidelines from which medical practice can evolve in a manner that enhances the care delivery experience and outcomes for patients and physicians alike, but also contributes to a resolution of the health care crisis.

The pressures causing the health care crisis have been distilled to a few characteristics, listed in Table 3.2. In some respects, this summary fails to capture the breadth and depth of each factor. Nonetheless, the summary manifestations do provide a general flavor of the challenges before physicians and medical groups. In a nutshell, the causal factors represent the following scenario: The medical field faces a knowledge explosion that threatens the sacred beliefs and relationships of physicians. No single physician can care for every patient and no physician can know all there is to know about medical care. The knowledge explosion undermines one-on-one relationships between patients and physicians. Specialization contributes to the demise of traditional patient-physician relationships. Patients are referred to specialists with whom they have never had a prior relationship. Thus, patients are thrust into a situation wherein they are expected to place great trust in a highly trained physician who essentially is a stranger.

Primary care gatekeepers discover that they are in conflict with the specialists to whom they refer patients. The primary physician is motivated to exercise control over the patient's care and otherwise

TABLE 3.2 Implications of Health Care Crisis Causal Factors for Medical Groups

Causal Factors	Summary Manifestations		
Excessive knowledge	• There is a sacred belief that medicine should be one-on-one. • There is an assumption that physicians can know all there is to know. • No single physician can care for every patient.		
Patient-physician relationships	• Speciailization has eroded patient's ability to maintain a trusting relationship with a physician. • Patients are referred to physicians with whom they have had no prior relationship. • Primary care gatekeepers are in conflict with specialists.	Drive	*Implications for Medical Groups* • Development of nontradtional practice structures • Integration of fundamental patient/ physician values about caring
Physicians	• Patient and physician expectations about the relationship are different. • Caring has been discarded for cutting-edge care. • Practice assumptions have changed.		
Medical terminology	• Technology has replaced judgment. • Diagnosis and treatment are mechanical. • Technology-based algorithms reduce the need for physicians.		

coordinate service delivery. However, the fragmented system transfers authority to the specialist who may prefer that different care modalities and treatment regimens transpire. In short, physician-patient relationships are compromised due to the increase in medical knowledge and the resulting shift to a referral-based delivery system. Physicians are discovering that the assumptions underlying their practices have changed enormously. Caring has been discarded. Cost and cutting-edge care are more important than caring. Meanwhile, patients have been led to expect that they will receive good results all of the time; that is, each medical encounter will resolve the medical malady. These pressures symbolize the rise of new expectations on the part of patients and physicians. The focus of each has changed.

Finally, the scenario conveyed in Table 3.2 involves the role of medical technology. Physicians are running headlong into an increasingly dominant imperative of medical technology. Diagnosis and treatment are more mechanical. Technology has replaced judgment and substituted algorithms. The result is a diminished need for physicians in many circumstances.

APPLICATIONS FOR MANAGERS

As managed care unfolds, there are distinct implications for medical groups. First, physicians must make intelligent choices about nontraditional practice structures. The historic practice options will eventually be discarded. Minor adjustments to the traditional practice patterns are proving insufficient to address the powerful set of pressures confronting physicians. The end result in that medical groups will be placed in the position of developing nontraditional practice patterns. Their focus will center on delivering the best care with the most confidence for the patient (and physician) and the least cost.

We want to emphasize that there is no one, best way, no cure-all or panacea for developing a nontraditional practice pattern. In many cases, medical groups will attempt to utilize gatekeepers as the coordinator for care delivery. This approach evolves naturally out of the family practice/general practitioner legacy from years past. Such an approach has its merits. However, it is possible to question whether this really generates a significant solution, or whether it simply delays the inevitable restructuring or reengineering necessary to comprehensively and systematically address the health care crisis factors.

It is essential to accentuate that fresh thinking should accompany the efforts by medical groups to develop nontraditional practice structures. For example, there may be great promise in using nonphysician providers in a triage approach to coordinate care. This has the advantage of building back into the system a single provider who knows the patient, who looks out for the patients, who develops a trusting relationship with the patient, who can interpret the system and care process for the patient, and whose services are considerably less expensive than those of physician gatekeepers. Whichever strategy is adopted, **physicians and medical groups should recognize that they are facing a situation wherein the tried and true no longer prevails, and where reliance on slight variations in the traditional themes will be insufficient to respond to the sweeping changes accompanying health care reform.**

The causal factors involving excessive knowledge, patient-physician relationships, physicians and medical technology have other implications for physicians and medical groups. There will be more pressure to devise practice settings that integrate fundamental patient and physician values about caring. Those medical groups that are able to incorporate a true sense of caring for patients will ultimately surface as desired providers. The challenge for medical groups is to integrate caring along with the other dominant characteristics needed for survival—low cost and high quality.

Medical groups that are committed to addressing the health care crisis will face another difficult necessity in tempering and balancing patient and physician expectations. Physician groups will need to reorient patients toward realistic expectations about the care they receive and the medical outcomes associated with that care. Medical groups must devise effective patient education programs that help clients understand not only the details surrounding the process of care, but also the actual deliverables that may be expected for any particular condition. Simultaneously, physicians themselves must attain a greater comfort level with the care outcomes that can be attained.

Finally, medical groups will need a new perspective on medical technology if they expect to negotiate the causal factors of the health care crisis. This begins by recognizing, rather than fighting, the value of medical technology and the rapid advancement in care delivery assists. If technology can facilitate the use of algorithms in care delivery, then astute medical groups must determine how they can use these algorithms to their advantage. If technology aids in replacing judgment during diagnosis and treatment, then astute medical groups will ascertain how they can capitalize accordingly. In short, **high-performing medical groups will be alert to ways in which they can utilize technology as an asset rather than viewing technology as a dysfunctional imperative.**

We have attempted to convey a new way of thinking that must be adopted by physicians and medical groups if they expect to successfully cope with the pressures for health care reform. Following chapters will provide further detail for an explicit agenda of strategies and tactics that medical groups and physicians can implement in order to take leadership and control over the health system and its perturbations.

REFERENCES

Alper, P. R. (1997, February 13). Learning to accentuate the positive in managed care. *New England Journal of Medicine, 336*(7), 508–509.

Azevedo, D. (1998, March 23). When the fighting's over will this practice still be standing? *Medical Economics,* 166–177.

Bindman, A. B., Grumbach, K., Uranizan, K., Jaffe, D., & Osmond, D. (1998, March 4). Selection and exclusion of primary care physicians by managed care organizations. *Journal of the American Medical Association, 279*(9), 675–679.

Blumenthal, D. (1996, Summer). Effects of market reforms on doctors and their patients. *Health Affairs, 15*(2), 170–84.

Bodenheimer, T., & Sullivan, K. (1998, April 12). How large employers are shaping the health care marketplace. *New England Journal of Medicine, 338*(14), 1003–1007.

Burns, L. (1996). Physicians and group practice: Balancing autonomy with market reality. *Journal of Ambulatory Care Management, 19*(3), 1–15.

Colby, D. C. (1997, November/December). Doctors and their discontents. *Health Affairs 16*(6), 112–114.

Deckard, G. J. (1995). Physician responses to a managed environment: A perceptual paradox. *Health Care Management Review, 20*(1), 40–46.

Freidson, E. (1972). The organization of medical practice. In H. E. Freeman, S. Levine, & L.G. Reeder (Eds.), *Handbook of medical sociology.* Englewood Cliffs, NJ: Prentice-Hall.

Goldfield, N. (1994). The looming fight over health care reform: What we can learn from past debates. *Health Care Management Review, 19*(3), 70–83.

Guptill Warren, M., Weitz, R., & Kulis, S. (1999). The impact of managed care on physicians. *Health Care Management Review, 24*(2), 44–56.

Hadley, J., & Mitchell, J. M. (1997, November/December). Effects of HMO market penetration on physicians' work effort and satisfaction. *Health Affairs.* 16(6), 99–111.

Herzlinger, R. E. (1998). The managerial revolution in the U.S. health care sector: Lessons from the U.S. economy. *Health Care Management Review,* 23(3), 19–29.

Heshmat, S. (1997). Commentary: Managed care and the relevant costs for pricing. *Health Care Management Review, 22*(1), 82–85.

How doctors can regain control of health care. (1996, May 13). *Medical Economics,* 178–201.

Hunt, R. E., & Newman, R. G. (1997). Medical knowledge overload: A disturbing trend for physicians. *Health Care Management Review, 22*(1), 70–75.

Johnson, E. (1995). The public's future perspective on managed care. *Health Care Management Review, 20*(2), 45–47.

Keeprews, D. (1995, Fall). The role of nurses in the new health care marketplace. *Health Affairs,* 280–281.

Kralewski, J. E., Rich, E. C., Bernhardt, T., Dowd, B., Feldman, R., & Johnson, C. (1998). The organizational structure of medical group practices in a managed care environment. *Health Care Management Review, 23*(2), 76–96.

Kuttner, R. (1998, May 21). Must good HMOs go bad? The search for checks and balances. Part I. *New England Journal of Medicine, 338*(21), 1558–1563.

National Opinion Research Center. (1995). *Survey of physicians about the Medicare program and fee schedule.* Washington, DC: Physician Payment Review Commission.

Pontes, M. C., & Pontes. N.M.H. (1997). Consumers' inferences about physician ability and accountability. *Health Care Management Review, 22*(2), 7–20.

Prince, T. R. (1998). A medical technology index for community hospitals. *Health Care Management Review, 23*(1), 52–63.

Starr, P. (1982). *The social transformation of American medicine.* New York: Basic Books.

Unland, J. J. (1995). The evolution of physician-directed managed care. *Journal of Health Care Finance, 22*(2), 42–56.

Walker, L. M. (1997, April 7). What it takes for small practices to succeed. *Medical Economics, 99, 104,* 113–116.

Walsh, A. M., & Borkowski, S. C. (1999). Cross-gender mentoring and career development in the health care industry. *Health Care Management Review, 24*(3), 7–17.

Woolhandler, S., & Himmelstein, D. V. (1995, Fall). The physician workforce delusion. *Health Affairs,* 279.

Chapter 4

A Patient-Centered
System of Care

Executive Summary

The statistics for patient satisfaction with managed care plans is rather dismal. Half of the consumers are disappointed with their service providers. This is not a very impressive finding for what once was the global epitome of medical care. In many respects, consumers have been left out of the equation in the restructuring of health care. Furthermore, as corporations drive hard bargains with managed care plans in order to provide low-cost coverage for their employees, they inadvertently minimize consumer choice. This only adds to the sense of dissatisfaction.

Medical groups must be ever attentive to patient relations if they expect to integrate consumers as active participants in care delivery and a contract for patient responsibility. Four strategies have particular importance in building better patient relations:

1. Assessing, monitoring and benchmarking care delivery;
2. Utilizing personal contracts for care to clarify patient and provider responsibilities;
3. Reorganizing facilities to enhance services; and
4. Developing electronic relations.

This chapter examines each of these strategies in detail. However, it is essential to recognize that any single approach is insufficient for articulating and executing innovation in health care delivery. These strategies form a basis from which embellishments create a unique and cutting edge for incorporating patients in care delivery.

A portion of this chapter was previously published as "Benchmarking Patient Relations Within Ambulatory Care: Lessons from a High-Risk Pregnancy Program," *Journal of Ambulatory Care Management*, 1999, 22(3), 58–71.

THE DEMISE OF PATIENT-PHYSICIAN RELATIONS

Almost half of all consumers are less than completely satisfied with their health plans (Jensen, 1996). Is it a case of the glass being half empty or half full? Perspective may not be all that important in this instance. What business can accept having almost half of its customers less than satisfied with its product or service? How long can such an organization survive? Should such a business be encouraged to survive or would it be better to hasten its demise at the hands of competitors? These are tough but relevant questions for health plans and providers in the health care system. Once protected from market forces, health care providers have experienced a startling reversal of fortune. Worse, the strategic responses by health providers have fallen far short of what customers—employers who pay for insurance benefits and employees who become patients—expect. Bruce Bradley, Director of Managed Care Plans for General Motors, argues that successful health plans will be those that put patients first while also driving down costs, enhancing provider satisfaction and improving quality (Bradley, 1997).

The American Association of Health Plans began an initiative to encourage members to center health care around consumers by putting them first. Most critics express skepticism about the ability of health plans to self-regulate their prevailing motives and interests (Havinghurst, 1997; Lee, 1997). Others express optimism that consumer purchasing power and quasi market forces will mean an end of the traditional health plan that dictated a very structured environment for care (Kleinke, 1998). The prospects for the future are more flexible and open health plans in which patients have choice in terms of coverage and access to physicians. The prospects are good for a physician-based system that does not propagate a contentious relation between patient and physician. In short, health plans will be forced to truly manage care rather than managing costs and attempting to control those who deliver care.

Figure 4.1 depicts the intersection of key pressures that are driving the health system toward patient-centered managed care and away from the nonsupportive traditions characterizing early health maintenance organizations. As Figure 4.1 suggests, most health plans are reaching, or have reached, the limits of incrementalism. There are diminishing returns from trying to squeeze out another penny in cost control, to get a service or product to market a few weeks earlier than

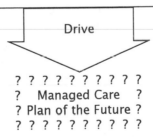

*Health care organizations are reaching
the limits of incrementalism:*
- Squeezing another penny out of costs;
- Getting a service or product to market a few weeks earlier;
- Responding to patient/customer needs a bit faster; and
- Capturing more market share and lives.

+

Managed cost is not equal to managed care:
- Physician income has been adversely affected.
- Care has not necessarily been managed (limited longitudinal information/proof).

+

The irreducible cost of care (that is, the basic cost of services needed to render quality care) has not been significantly affected.

+

Choice matters:
- People value choice and choice increases satisfaction with managed care.
- People need information to make appropriate choices.

Drive

? ? ? ? ? ? ? ? ? ?
?   Managed Care   ?
? Plan of the Future ?
? ? ? ? ? ? ? ? ? ?

Figure 4.1   The Pressure for Patient-Centered Managed Care

a competitor, to respond to patient or customer needs a bit faster, or to capture more market share and lives. In the final analysis, health maintenance organizations have done little to manage health, although they have tried conscientiously to manage costs. As a result, health care insurance premiums have been somewhat contained, physician income has been decreased, and limited evidence has surfaced that health care outcomes have improved. Add to these trends the fact that the basic cost of health services—the fundamental base needed to render quality care—has not been significantly affected, and consumers are seeking more choice and more information to make intelligent choices (Davis, Collins, Schoen, & Morris, 1995).

The inability of some health maintenance organizations to successfully cope with the pressures listed in Figure 4.1 has resulted in a shake-out in the industry. From a purely economic perspective, this implies a more efficient market. However, from the consumer's perspective, this situation presents several ominous indications (Bailit, 1997). Fewer suppliers (that is, health plans) concentrates power in the hands of fewer providers. In 1996, the result was 40 percent of U.S. hospitals engaging in some variety of merger or acquisition activity (*Modern Healthcare,* 1996). The problem is aggravated because consolidation has left insurance companies and investor-owned businesses in control. This seriously threatens patient support and physician-patient relations (Yarmolinsky, 1995).

The Sanctity of Physician-Patient Relations

The doctor-patient relationship is one of the most sacred medical ideals. It is considered the fundamental basis and cornerstone of good practice. All other factors aside, a rewarding doctor-patient relationship is considered a prerequisite for good care. Although patients simply desire a good relationship with a physician, doctors believe a strong relationship is crucial for good care. While health care seeks to achieve good doctor-patient relationships, a rewarding relationship seems to be increasingly elusive. In the past, good relationships just seemed to happen without any particular effort on the part of either doctor or patient. With all the scientific progress in medicine, why are we losing this cornerstone of medical care? What has changed and why has change occurred? Can we bring it back? What exactly was the basis of a rewarding relationship and, if we cannot bring it back, is there any kind of reasonable substitute? By attempting to answer these questions we can better understand why the health care delivery system is headed toward disaster.

A strong doctor-patient relationship is often powerful medicine. The confidence and feeling that there is someone who can help to make you well is really the basis of a rewarding doctor-patient relationship (Mechanic & Schlesinger, 1996). In analyzing this thought further, a number of prerequisites for a rewarding relationship are apparent. First, the patient must know and trust the doctor. Second, the patient must have a sufficient choice of physicians to be able to find someone he or she likes and trusts. Third, the doctors must know and feel that they have a good relationship with patients. Fourth, the patient must feel that when help is needed, the doctor will be available (Tudor, Riley, & Ingber, 1998). It helps if one doctor can take care of most or all of the patient's problems. However, if referral to another physician is necessary, the patient's doctor should be available for sympathy and support.

This simple concept functioned well in the past because, except for surgical operations, it was about all the doctor could do. Doctors' primary focus was caring, giving assurance and hoping for a good result. Their minds were not burdened with the dual problems of providing a relationship and providing highly scientific medical care. The concept also worked well because patients did not and could not necessarily expect good results. Timely recovery was often in the hands of a higher power.

The Prospects for Physician-Patient Relationships

Where do all of these changes lead? The basic concept of a rewarding doctor-patient relationship is valid. It is necessary for good care and for patient confidence, as suggested in Table 4.1. Bodenheimer and colleagues (1998) demonstrated that cost of care and affiliation with a physician are the primary factors determining care system choices. Several years ago, organized medicine tried to address the problem of building physician-patient relations by promoting the primary physician concept. This idea was an attempt to give patients some security in working within the health care system. Each patient had a primary physician who provided security, enabled the patient to utilize a complicated system, and provided basic care to the point that a specialist was necessary. Family practice residencies were started, and many medical school graduates subsequently entered family practice.

TABLE 4.1   The New Reality of Consumer Preferences

Factors Determining Care System Choices

- Price
  - 26 percent of health plan enrollees switched to a cheaper plan when the monthly premium for their own plan rose by $10.
- Existing family physician
- Location
- On-site parking
- Gender of the doctor
- Recommendations of family and friends
- Report cards on provider quality of care

Source: T. Bodenheimer et al. (1998). How large employers are shaping the health care marketplace. *New England Journal of Medicine. 338*(14): 1003–7.

The thrust for family practice has intensified in larger clinics and health maintenance organizations where patients must have a primary physician. Initially, it was hoped that the entire family would be taken care of by one family physician just as in times past. The physician would render care until the point at which she or he as an individual wanted the help of a specialist. Unfortunately, the idea has not worked out as well as planned if the implementation is critically analyzed. There are several problems from patients' points of view.

There is still the problem of choosing a physician that fits the patient's personality so that a rewarding relationship can develop. At one time, patients could visit several doctors in solo practice and choose a primary provider. In a health maintenance organization or other managed care plan, the patient can still interview several physicians; but the ones that are rejected may be the next to see the patient if there is a problem at night or on the weekend. Often the most likable and popular primary physicians have a full panel of patients and will not take new patients.

If physicians are popular, and therefore busy, it may be difficult to get an appointment that is convenient for the patient. It almost seems that convenience for the managed care plan is more important than convenience for either patient or doctor. In addition, a patient with an ongoing problem who has seen an appropriate specialist for the problem (with a good relationship and good results) may be forced to change to a new primary physician who does not know about either the patient or the problem. Finally, the patient with a chronic problem may suspect that further complicated care is being discouraged—feeling, in effect, a subtle form of rationing.

As the health delivery system evolved, doctors were also encountering problems. When health care became more like a business and costs were important, doctors were encouraged to see more patients. Sometimes, primary physicians felt they had an excessively large panel of patients that prevented them from providing the best quality care. There was also an enormous increase in paperwork to ensure that patients did not make successful self-referrals to specialists; that is, that patients contacted the primary physician in all cases and that the primary physician made the proper referrals. Usually, there were guidelines for referral and guidelines for surgical operations so that primary providers were not able to refer when they individually felt it was desirable. Within these guidelines there were quotas and bonuses or fines for not being within the prescribed limits.

The primary physician, thus, has a gatekeeper function to manage patients that sometimes conflicts with his or her own desires to refer to a specialist (Forrest & Reid, 1997). With regard to a rewarding relationship, the gatekeeper function is absolutely contrary to a good outcome. **Gatekeeping is not in the best interest of either patient or doctor because it implies that the physician will prevent patients from obtaining something they want.** Primary physicians may also find they are in conflict with specialists who think an earlier referral would have been more desirable.

There are problems for the system as well. The family practice concept became fragmented at the start. Three specialties were able to provide primary physicians: family practice, internal medicine and pediatrics. In some areas, obstetrics-gynecologists were primary physicians for women. Everyone in the family, therefore, had the potential of having a different primary physician. The system still has the problem that patients may not have a rewarding relationship with a doctor and, hence, are angry with the system. Basically, the family practice idea has not been able to satisfy the prerequisites for a rewarding relationship in the arena of modern health care.

THE RIGHT TO CHOOSE

Consumers are facing a very real predicament in developing rewarding relations with physicians given the progress in managed care and gatekeeping. However, the situation is aggravated by the decreasing ability to control which plans an employer offers as a health benefit. Employers are shopping on behalf of dozens, hundreds or thousands of employees, not for a single individual. Thus, there is a strong probability that employees will discover that the managed care plans available to them do not include their family physician on the physician panels. The result is reduction in choice for the consumer and, consequently, reduction in satisfaction with health care coverage and delivery. Light (1996) observes that patient ability to choose can be inadvertently usurped by employers when they select managed care plans with whom they contract for employee care.

Further insights on the right of patients to choose their family practitioners and its demise under managed care are presented in Figure 4.2. Bodenheimer and colleagues (1998) trace the predicament in consumer choice back to 1988 when Allied Signal (now Honeywell) consolidated all health care benefits into a contract with Cigna for health maintenance organization coverage. Allied Signal enrolled approximately 80,000 employees under the Cigna banner and, in the process, negotiated a three-year cap on the costs of health insurance coverage. From Allied Signal's perspective, it was ensuring access to low-cost and quality care for employees while simultaneously saving millions of dollars through the negotiated contract.

Although Allied Signal was the prime beneficiary from its decision to limit health coverage options, the ultimate impact for employee choice was adverse. Unless an employee's physician was part of the Cigna system, the employee was not able to receive Allied Signal coverage for health care services rendered. While this was a distinct imposition for Allied Signal employees, the ramification for employers and employees nationwide were tremendous. Which right was more important—the right of the employer to negotiate lower health costs through contractual arrangements with one or more insurers, or the right of employees to maintain their relationship with specific physicians? How could employees protect their rights to choose given these actions of corporations that had vastly larger amounts of resources to impose their decisions (Annas, 1997)?

The implications from Allied Signal's actions were soon apparent. By the late 1990s, more than 50 million people received health care through employer-sponsored HMOs and another 50 million people were enrolled in preferred provider organizations (PPOs). These facts indicated that corporations moved swiftly toward the Allied Signal model by restricting choice through contractual arrangement with

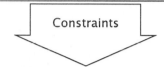

The Revolution

In 1988, Allied-Signal canceled all health care arrangements for 80,000 employees and enrolled them into Cigna's HMO plans:
- Allied-Signal negotiated a three-year cap on costs.
- Allied-Signal saved millions of dollars.

Constraints

Consumer Choice

- Now, more than 50 million people receive health care through employer-sponsored HMOs; another 50 million are enrolled in preferred provider organizations.
- Almost 50 percent of employees in large companies have no choice of health plans; 91 percent of employees in small companies have no choice.
- Unless a corporation has thousands of employees, it has limited incentive or staff to direct-contract with providers.
- Corporations encounter limited switching costs; the burden falls on employees and their families.
- One-half of all enrollees report switching health plans in a three-year period; 73 percent report the switch was involuntary.

FIGURE 4.2   Consumer Choice Constrained by Corporate Control

Source: T. Bodenheimer et al. (1998). How large employers are shaping the health care marketplace. *New England Journal of Medicine.* 338(14): 1003–7.

managed care plans. As a result, almost 50 percent of employees in large companies had no choice of health plan while almost 91 percent of all employees in small companies had no choice of health plan whatsoever. Thus, it is easy to argue that the one bearing the brunt of rising health costs was not the corporate sector but, rather, the employees. Corporations reap the reward of lower health costs at the expense of employee choice of physician.

The problem is exacerbated by the limited incentive corporations have to remain with any single health provider. Corporations are primarily looking out for the bottom line, although they will express enormous rhetoric about the importance of quality of care that health plans must document when the corporation assesses options for employee health coverage. In reality, corporations do not invest sufficiently in the level of staffing it takes to thoroughly assess health plan options. Thus, corporations are susceptible to marketing efforts by the health plans. Furthermore, corporations have very insignificant switching costs—that is, the costs associated with the change in contract from one health plan to another. The burden falls upon the employees and their families who may have to terminate their relationship with a physician or physicians and establish new relations within another health plan. The magnitude of this problem is enormous. One-half of all enrollees in health plans report switching plans in a three-year period. Seventy-three percent of these individuals indicate that the switch was involuntary.

Wilensky (1995) has speculated that this switching phenomenon, due to corporate and large organization affiliation with health plans, produces more change in the health system with negative consequences than under the traditional system. She predicts that continuity of care suffers as well as consumer satisfaction. Her proposition is well grounded. How can health care be managed when patients are constantly switching physicians? No sooner does a physician begin to understand the medical needs of patients and their families than they are gone and enrolled in another health plan where the process starts all over again. This is very inefficient for the health care system and deleterious for achieving any intelligent form of managed care. Primary care of fundamental health issues requires years to reach efficacy. This continuity and methodical intervention is difficult, if not impossible, to attain when patients and physicians are constantly being shuffled due to corporate interests for controlling short-term health costs that improve the current year's financial profile.

TOWARD IMPROVED PHYSICIAN-PATIENT RELATIONS

The effort to attain improved physician-patient relations and a patient-centered system of care will require a shift in thinking about service delivery. There are several strategies that medical groups can consider in building better patient relations. First, medical groups must remain attuned to the preferences of patients and their satisfaction with those service delivery efforts. This can be accomplished through monitoring, assessment and benchmarking programs. Second, medical groups can utilize personal contracts for care to clarify patient and provider responsibilities. Third, medical groups can reorganize facilities to enhance services. Finally, medical groups can move toward electronic relations for consumers of the future. Each of these strategies will be discussed.

Assessing, Monitoring and Benchmarking Care Delivery

A patient-centered care delivery effort must incorporate a significant devotion to assessing and monitoring patient perceptions on the quality of care. In short, how can a medical group lay claim to delivering high-quality care unless it is able to provide evidence of its outcomes (Shortell, Gillies, & Anderson, 1994)? Furthermore, for its internal applications, assessment of the care delivery process and outcomes are integral to benchmarking by medical groups. Continuous quality improvement depends on establishing verifiable baselines and comparing subsequent performance with those baselines as well as benchmarks of best practices by other medical groups (Corrigan, 1995). Patient-centered care assumes that medical groups will invest substantially and continuously in assessment, monitoring and benchmarking. The art and science of these activities have evolved considerably in corporate applications. A reinvented care delivery system can benefit from these techniques.

Ford, Bach and Fottler (1997) reviewed the various methods of measuring patient satisfaction in health care. They separated the assessment methodologies into two groups: qualitative techniques and quantitative techniques. Although Ford, Bach and Fottler reviewed these assessment tools with patient satisfaction in mind, it is clear that the methodologies have much broader application for evaluating relations with diverse internal and external stakeholders. For example, a medical group might use these tools for measuring the attitudes of nurses to a change in organization, or to ascertain the insights technicians might have for enhancing patients' satisfaction with treatment. Measurement might be used to gain insights on solving problems just as well as discovering how well or poorly services have been delivered in the eyes of the recipients.

Table 4.2 presents qualitative measures that can give medical group management and staff information on the service delivery process and its outcomes. According to Ford, Bach and Fottler, two groups of individuals are positioned to observe operations and the

TABLE 4.2   Qualitative Techniques for Assessing Service Delivery

Advantages and Disadvantages of Various Qualitative Management Techniques For Measuring Patient Service Quality

Management Techniques	Advantages	Disadvantages
Management observation	• Management knows business, policies and procedures • No inconvenience to patient • Opportunity to recover from service failure • Opportunity to obtain detailed patient feedback • Opportunity to identify service delivery problems • Minimal incremental cost for data gathering	• Management presence may influence service providers • Lacks statistical validity and reliability • Objective observation requires specialized training • Employees disinclined to report problems they created • Management may be unfamiliar with processes and customers
Employment feedback programs	• Employees have knowledge of service delivery obstacles • Patients volunteer service experience information to employees • No inconvenience to patients • Opportunity to recover from service failure • Employee empowerment improves morale • Opportunity to collect detailed patient feedback • Minimal incremental cost for data gathering and documentation	• Objective observation requires specialized training • Employees disinclined to report problems they created
Work teams and quality circles	• Develop employee awareness of management's strong commitment to service quality • Develop an understanding and appreciation of how each employee can directly influence service quality	• Must have employees who can handle responsibilities of empowerment • Team must act cohesively and work together • Necessary communication among team members takes large amounts of time

TABLE 4.2 Continued

Advantages and Disadvantages of Various Qualitative Management Techniques For Measuring Patient Service Quality

Management Techniques	Advantages	Disadvantages
Focus groups	• Through empowerment, improve employee morale, productivity, efficiency, effectiveness and patient satisfaction • Team working together conveys confidence and competence to patients • Opportunities to collect detailed patient feedback • Opportunity to recover from service failure • Qualitative analysis helps to focus managers on problem areas • Other problems may surface during discussions • Suggest that facility is interested in patient's opinions of service quality	• May only identify symptoms and not core service delivery problems • Feedback limited to small group of customers • Information representative with repeat sampling • Recollection of specific service encounter details may be lost • One group member may dominate or bias discussion • Inconvenience necessitates incentives for participation • High cost of properly trained focus group leader • Information may be withheld due to fear of disapproval by others • May not be representative samples of the patient population

Source: Adapted from R. C. Ford, S. A. Bach, & M. D. Fottler. (1997). Methods of measuring patient satisfaction in health care organizations. *Health Care Management Review, 22*(2), 74–89.

results from service delivery—management and staff. Simply in the course of performing their jobs, people observe system dysfunctions and successes. They are able to observe patient reactions to the structure, process and outcomes of care. They are able to observe how patients interact with clinicians and nonclinicians. The proximity of management and staff to service delivery means that they may serve as useful conduits of information. However, Table 4.2 reviews some of the disadvantages of using observation by organizational members as a means to assess and monitor performance. Staff members can lack objectivity due to their time with and experience in an organization. They are predisposed to various interpretations of service delivery in view of this experience. Staff members also are usually not trained to observe in an objective and systematic fashion.

A third form of organizational means of assessing and monitoring performance is the quality circle and work team. Quality circles are normally comprised of six to eight members with the assignment of solving problems or instilling improvements within operations. As part of the continuous quality improvement process, there is a well-defined methodology for utilizing quality circles. There are many advantages of quality circles, but they are especially useful in integrating staff in the systematic collection of data, data assessment and interpretation, and problem resolution. The primary downside of quality circles and continuous quality improvement in medical groups has been the tendency for physicians to not embrace the process.

The fourth form of qualitative approach for assessing and monitoring information is focus groups. Internal and external participants can form a focus group that typically has 10 participants who express opinions about service delivery. A facilitator directs the discussion of the focus group to gain critical views of performance and suggestions for improvement. The primary downside of a focus group is the inability to include large proportions of patients (or employees) in the sample. If a health plan has 100,000 members and the plan is interested in hearing about the performance of the women's health program, the focus groups can be used to test various assumptions about items that might be included on a survey questionnaire that would be distributed to all female patients. However, it is unlikely that focus group feedback would be considered a representative sample.

Balancing the qualitative methods for assessing, monitoring and benchmarking performance are the quantitative techniques shown in Table 4.3. The predominant advantages of quantitative approaches are their ability to assess large samples through broad dissemination and the accuracy of analysis through quantitative methods. Health care organizations have tended to use comment cards, mail surveys and telephone interviews in collecting data. On-site, structured personal interviews are less commonplace due to the labor involved. This technique can also be viewed as a qualitative methodology. Mystery shoppers, like on-site personal interviews, can also be viewed as a qualitative tool depending on the degree of structure in the questions, issues or observations comprising the assessment.

Mail surveys, or surveys that are widely distributed to a large sample of respondents, are a prevalent technique for acquiring information. Although Ford, Bach and Fottler (1997) express the value of beginning performance assessment with qualitative techniques, the quantitative approaches are probably more widely used even among those just initiating quality improvement programs. Sidebar 4.1 provides one example of a survey application in a mental health setting. Ford, Bach and Fottler (1997) also express the opinion that health care organizations should prudently select the combination of quantitative and qualitative techniques that will be used in assessing, monitoring and benchmarking performance. In other words, **there is no panacea for assessing patient satisfaction, quality of care or performance benchmarks.** Even the existing instrumentation, such as for quality of care, may need modification in order to fit with the particular needs of a group practice.

The promising reality for programs that assess, monitor and benchmark care delivery is the extensive number of techniques, tried and proven, from which to draw in the continuous improvement effort. Not every physician or medical group has knowledge of every technique or application. They do not need in-depth knowledge because this can be acquired from external resources at reasonable cost. What cannot be acquired externally is a commitment to developing sound quality improvement programs. This inspiration can only be derived internally. High-performing medical groups move beyond the rhetoric and details of assessment. They become obsessed with performance improvement that is guided by reliable analysis.

TABLE 4.3 Quantitative Techniques for Assessing Service Delivery

Advantages and Disadvantages of Various Quantitative Management Techniques For Measuring Patient Service Quality

Management Techniques	Advantages	Disadvantages
Comment cards	▪ Suggest that facility is interested in patients' opinions of service quality ▪ Opportunity to recover from service failure ▪ Minimal incremental cost for data gathering ▪ Moderate cost	▪ Self-selected sample of patients not statistically representative ▪ Comments generally reflect extreme patient dissatisfaction or extreme satisfaction
Mail surveys	▪ Ability to gather representative and valid samples of targeted patients ▪ Opportunity to recover from service failure ▪ Patients can reflect on their service experience ▪ Suggest that facility is interested in patients' opinions of service quality ▪ Allow comparisons of patient satisfaction by department and patient demographics	▪ Recollection of specific service encounter details may be lost ▪ Other service experiences may bias responses because of time lag ▪ Inconvenience necessitates incentives for participants ▪ Cost to gather representative sample may be high ▪ Potential problems with the wording of questions
Onsite personal interviews	▪ Opportunity to collect detailed patient feedback ▪ Opportunity to recover from service failure ▪ Ability to gather representative and valid samples of targeted patients ▪ Suggest that facility is interested in patients' opinions of service quality	▪ May not be representative sample of patients ▪ Recollection of specific service encounter details may be lost ▪ Other service experiences may bias responses because of time lag ▪ Respondents tend to give socially desirable responses

TABLE 4.3 Continued

Advantages and Disadvantages of Various Quantitative Management Techniques For Measuring Patient Service Quality

Management Techniques	Advantages	Disadvantages
Telephone interviews	▪ Opportunity to collect detailed patient feedback ▪ Ability to gather representative and valid sample of targeted patients ▪ Opportunity to recover from service failure ▪ Suggest that facility is interested in patients' opinions of service quality	▪ Inconvenience necessitates incentives for participants ▪ Cost is moderate to high ▪ Individuals tend to find telephone call intrusive ▪ Difficult to contact people at work; inconvenient at home ▪ Costs of skilled interviewers and valid instrument are high ▪ May not generate a representative cross-section of patients
Mystery shoppers	▪ Consistent and unbiased feedback ▪ Can focus on specific situations ▪ No inconveniences to patient ▪ Opportunity to collect detailed feedback ▪ Allows measurement of training program effectiveness	▪ Snapshot of isolated encounters may be statistically invalid ▪ Cost is moderate to high ▪ Not applicable to all clinical areas (for example, surgery) ▪ Ethical concerns

Source: Adapted from R. C. Ford, S. A. Bach, & M. D. Fottler. (1997). Methods of measuring patient satisfaction in health care organization. *Health Care Management Review, 22*(2),74–89.

Sidebar 4.1
Client Satisfaction in a Mental Health Organization

A large, national mental health care organization collected client satisfaction data using a 21-item survey instrument. The instrument measured:

- Overall satisfaction with the client-therapist relationship;
- Empathy demonstrated by the therapist;
- Treatment planning by the therapist;
- Fit or match between client and therapist;
- Satisfaction with number of visits/sessions delivered; and
- Satisfaction with the access and coordination of care.

The preceding constructs were created from specific survey items. Each item was assessed according to a 5-point Likert scale with 1 = excellent (highest level of satisfaction) and 5 = poor (lowest level of satisfaction).

The objective of this assessment was to improve client satisfaction. By evaluating various dimensions of satisfaction, the mental health organization would ascertain where to place greatest emphasis in continuous quality improvement efforts.

The following results surfaced in the study:

Constructs	*% of Respondents Assessing Highest Ratings*
Overall Satisfaction	
▪ To what extent has our program met your needs?	81.5
▪ Have the services received helped you to deal more effectively with your problems?	90.4
▪ In an overall, general sense, how satisfied are you with the services you received?	86.1
▪ If you were to seek help again, would you come back to our program?	88.2
Empathy	
▪ Your therapist listened closely to you	83.7
▪ Your therapist understood your problem and how you felt about it	76.0

continued

Constructs	% of Respondents Assessing Highest Ratings
Treatment Planning	
▪ Your therapist described how you would work together (your treatment plan)	66.4
Therapist Match	
▪ How satisfied were you with the match between the therapist's skills/specialty and your concerns?	72.5
Duration	
▪ How satisfied were you with the number of appointments you have received?	70.1
Access and Coordination	
How satisfied were you with:	
▪ The ease with which you got through on the telephone	71.7
▪ The time you waited between calling for your first appointment and the appointment time you received	73.7
▪ The time you waited between appointments after your first one	77.4
▪ The convenience of appointment times for your schedule	75.4
▪ The telephone and office staff's courtesy and responsiveness	73.5
▪ The pleasantness of the physical environment	72.5
▪ The amount of paperwork you were asked to complete	76.8
▪ The coordination of services among the therapist, those making your appointments, and others involved in your care	70.7

The analysis indicated that the single, most powerful predictor of the highest client satisfaction is the match or fit between client and therapist. With this finding, the mental health organization designed tactics to improve the client-therapist match.

Source: Adapted from B. L. Ingram & R. S. Chung. (1997). Client satisfaction data and quality improvement planning in managed mental health organizations. *Health Care Management Review, 22*(3), 40–52.

Benchmarking Patient Relations

Driven by the ever-tightening constraints of managed care, health care providers are highly cognizant of the need to progressively improve service delivery. Consequently, health care organizations are devoting considerable attention to quality improvement methodologies that utilize benchmarks. They recognize that measurable performance gains are one ingredient for successfully responding to pressure for lower cost, higher quality and improved access. In the past, quality assurance and utilization management programs in hospitals and other intensive care settings provided a convenient platform for the evolution of inpatient quality control programs. Unfortunately, providers in medical group environments often lacked these historic programs to use as a foundation for process and outcome improvements. However, there is a positive side to the relatively recent development of quality improvement processes in outpatient or ambulatory settings. Many health care providers are now focusing on innovative ways to enhance performance (Chesanow, 1998).

Benchmarking has become a metaphor for performance improvement among health care providers. Whether a home health agency, medical group, hospice, urgent care center or other genre of outpatient care delivery, there is great interest in understanding causal factors and variables that, when manipulated, might improve performance. Because performance is a complex concept with many manifestations, it is understandable that incremental gains in measuring performance and comparing performance to internal and external benchmarks is a focus of most quality improvement programs.

Clinical, fiscal, personnel, plant and equipment, patient and a vast array of other performance variables demand careful examination and management in today's financial environment. Nonetheless, there are often few reliable sources of comparable information. Providers usually settle on experimenting with internal measures while seeking benchmarks that offer a comparative basis to contemplate trends. Usually, the available cross-industry or cross-organizational performance benchmarks possess significant limitations that render them useful only as gross indicators. Throughout these settings, health care providers are challenged to establish reliable benchmarks that help to progressively direct operations toward higher levels of sustainable goal attainment.

Benchmarking is especially problematic in the area of patient relations. Customer and guest relations have traditionally been overlooked as critical care delivery issues by the health system. Now that patients expect more than just low-cost and high-quality care, there is a scramble to improve patients' or clients' experiences with health care organizations. Unfortunately, there is a serious shortfall in the availability of comparative statistics, measures and other benchmarking in outpatient and inpatient settings alike.

Following is a brief review of several of the significant barriers to benchmarking patient relations in health care organizations, especially medical clinics, and several strategies for improvement. Lessons from the Lovelace Health System's High Risk Pregnancy Program are discussed in exemplifying how benchmarking can encourage innovation and enhanced performance. The Lovelace Health System is located in Albuquerque, N.M. It is centered around a 180,000-member health maintenance organization. Care is delivered at a main medical center supported by eight satellite clinics within metropolitan Albuquerque. The main clinic is integrated with a 225-bed hospital. Managed care is provided through the Lovelace Health Plan.

A Benchmark for Patient-Physician Relations

The dilemma confronting patient relations with providers evolved from a benchmark established 50 years ago when each patient went to one doctor and a close relationship was formed. Over time, hospitals, specialists and insurance companies evolved in complexity, creating a situation in which patients interacted with a system rather than with a single physician. This historic benchmark and its impact on patient relations are shown in Figure 4.3.

Primary care physicians have two medical functions: to care for patients as long as possible and to triage patients to specialists when it is mandatory. These benchmarks of care are increasingly compromised in the managed care environment. Triage essentially means that the patient gets to the right place in a complex system. Contemporary care delivery often misses the mark in this regard. Even the primary physician-patient relationship does not work well in modern health delivery systems because most doctors sign out to other physicians at night. Thus, if patients need help at night or on weekends, they may have to relate to someone they do not know and may not like. As a result, not all aspects of the traditional doctor-patient relationship (benchmark) exist at the present. The patient

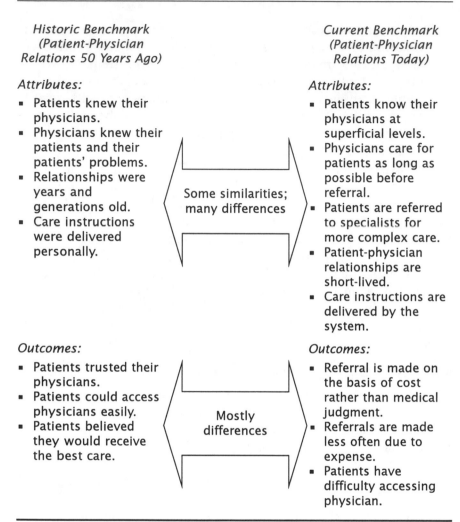

*Historic Benchmark
(Patient-Physician
Relations 50 Years Ago)*

*Current Benchmark
(Patient-Physician
Relations Today)*

Attributes:
- Patients knew their physicians.
- Physicians knew their patients and their patients' problems.
- Relationships were years and generations old.
- Care instructions were delivered personally.

Some similarities; many differences

Attributes:
- Patients know their physicians at superficial levels.
- Physicians care for patients as long as possible before referral.
- Patients are referred to specialists for more complex care.
- Patient-physician relationships are short-lived.
- Care instructions are delivered by the system.

Outcomes:
- Patients trusted their physicians.
- Patients could access physicians easily.
- Patients believed they would receive the best care.

Mostly differences

Outcomes:
- Referral is made on the basis of cost rather than medical judgment.
- Referrals are made less often due to expense.
- Patients have difficulty accessing physician.

FIGURE 4.3   The Demise of Rewarding Patient-Provider Relations

may not have a relationship with the doctor; the patient cannot see a specialist if desired; and, in some instances, the physician cannot refer the patient to a specialist when the primary physician thinks it is necessary for the best care. As indicated in Figure 4.3, there are some similarities but many more differences when looking at patient-physician relations today compared with the benchmark set 50 years ago.

Establishing a New Benchmark

Several new benchmarks must be met with respect to patient-physician relationships for care delivery to evolve (Asher, 1997):

1. Patients should be able to call a provider who has a previous professional relationship with the patient. The patient can call any time of the day or night, 24 hours a day, 7 days a week, 365 days a year.

2. The patient should know, like, and be comfortable with the contact person. If the primary contact person is not available, a secondary person, whom the patient has previously met, will respond.

3. The contact person will have some knowledge of the patient (ostensibly accessed and managed through a computer), and if the primary contact person answers, he or she would know the patient as an individual.

4. The contact person will have sufficient authority to ensure that the patient is seen on an emergency basis (if necessary) by the most experienced person for the patient's problem.

As suggested in Figure 4.4, these new benchmarks are similar to those that were met by patient-physician relations before each patient had to interrelate with a complex system.

The four benchmarks can be achieved through case managers and, in the process, case managers can assist in addressing several difficult problems (Singleton & Kilburn, 1995). They solve the relationship problem between each patient and the system. They provide a means for ensuring around-the-clock contact with someone the patient knows and who knows the patient. They also provide effective triage to those with maximum expertise for the patient's current problem. Case managers help to minimize the gatekeeper concept. If implemented correctly by providing case managers sufficient authority, administrative costs can be reduced (Micheletti & Shala, 1995). In essence, the new benchmark becomes the motivation for improved patient relations.

A New Benchmark for Patient-Physician Relations

The case management model using nonphysicians for triage embodies an innovative concept and benchmark for medical care.

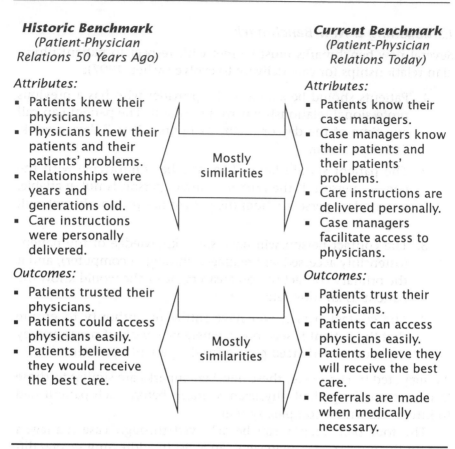

Historic Benchmark
(Patient-Physician
Relations 50 Years Ago)

Attributes:

- Patients knew their physicians.
- Physicians knew their patients and their patients' problems.
- Relationships were years and generations old.
- Care instructions were personally delivered.

Outcomes:

- Patients trusted their physicians.
- Patients could access physicians easily.
- Patients believed they would receive the best care.

Current Benchmark
(Patient-Physician
Relations Today)

Attributes:

- Patients know their case managers.
- Case managers know their patients and their patients' problems.
- Care instructions are delivered personally.
- Case managers facilitate access to physicians.

Outcomes:

- Patients trust their physicians.
- Patients can access physicians easily.
- Patients believe they will receive the best care.
- Referrals are made when medically necessary.

Mostly similarities

Mostly similarities

FIGURE 4.4 Rebuilding Patient-Provider Relations through Case Management

Case management separates the triage function from the care function. The person who performs triage for the patient in a medical group does not provide actual care, and the person who provides care does not usually perform the triage function. At first, this care delivery protocol may trouble physicians who have traditionally had triage authority. However, if physicians objectively assess the current situation, much of the triage they currently perform (that is, determining whom the patient can see and when) is being delegated to support staff.

The case management approach sets a new benchmark for physician productivity by relieving them from trying to maintain an all-encompassing, primary relationship with patients while simultaneously trying to hold down the cost of care. Close patient relations may represent a goal that doctors sincerely desire, but it is a role they can no longer effectively provide. The case management model relieves doctors from misallocating time away from actual health care to perform triage and therefore raises physician productivity while lowering costs.

The case management model also sets a new benchmark for cost-effectiveness because case managers are usually paid one-third or one-fourth as much as a physician in the primary care role. For most patients, case managers can make a very effective referral to the appropriate doctor with the maximum expertise for the current problem. In many instances, this will be a specialist with whom the patient has an ongoing relationship for a past problem. The case management model provides an ongoing relationship with someone the patient has chosen, knows and trusts. This person acts as an interface with a medical group and enables the patient to quickly see a provider who has maximum expertise for the problem. If the model works effectively, the patient will see the case manager as an advocate. Because the care function is separated from the relationship and triage function, there should be no conflict of interest (between gatekeeping and care rationing) for the case managers.

Patient Satisfaction through Personal Contracts

Physicians and medical groups should also consider the viability of person contracts with patients as a means to improve quality, efficiency and patient satisfaction. Evidence is accumulating that a personal contract for each patient might assist in promoting understanding of the actual condition, modifying patients' denial and improving satisfaction with care (Grandinetti, 1996). Patients would receive full knowledge about their responsibilities before agreeing to a contract. By entering into a personal contract, some of the denial would be alleviated because patients would be better informed about care. The concept of a contract is based on the fact that when patients have a sudden, severe illness (for example, a heart attack) they learn all they can about the condition, accept a realistic prognosis and often entirely change their behavior in a positive manner to assist recovery. A written contract might assist patients' motivation to understand their health and to change behavior without the shock of a severe illness (see Figure 4.5).

The Personal Contract Concept

- Patients receive accurate, substantive information about their condition.
- Options for treatment are defined.
- Probable results from treatment are classified.
- Lifestyle impact from care will be delineated.
- Patient behavior responsibilities are identified.

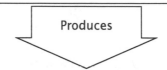

Produces

Enhanced Patient Satisfaction

- Better understanding by patient;
- Realistic patient expectations;
- Altered patient behavior; and
- Alleviation of denial.

FIGURE 4.5   Patient Satisfaction from a Personal Contract
for Health

A contract would affect all subsequent care and would have a distinctive, positive impact in controlling costs and raising productivity. Decisions on whether or not to have an operation; the probable results of medication; what aspects of lifestyle should be changed; what results can be expected (with and without the proposed changes); and how patients should behave after a procedure/operation represent only a few of the parameters surrounding a personal contract. There would be multiple benefits for raising provider productivity and for reducing costs. If patients signed the contract, they would take more responsibility as a partner in managing care, and the contract would be strong stimulus for them to change behavior in a positive fashion.

The concept of an individual contract for health is elemental to a reinvented health care system and high-performing medical groups. If the goal of delivering the right care at the right time with kindness and caring at the most effective cost is to be reached, it is obvious that each patient must understand his or her own health and act as a full partner in reaching the goal. With a personal contract, patients will receive accurate, substantive information about their condition, arrive at a real understanding of what this information means, and internalize any recommendations for the future. This process cannot be accomplished in a short office visit with a physicians, but case managers could accomplish the task. It might even be effectively achieved in a group session involving several patients with the same problems.

The patient would be presented with a contract of what the provider recommends and what intervention will occur as far as clinical treatment. The contract also spells out what the patient should do under the circumstances. The contract would either be signed or rejected. If rejected, it would make no difference in the care received except that the results might not be as favorable. The patient would be informed that because of his or her decision, optimum health care cannot necessarily be provided. **A formal contract that is either accepted or rejected will promote better understanding and should solve one of the most critical problems in health care: expectations.** At one time, all patients were confronted with their mortality because death was a visible experience. Everyone knew someone who had died prematurely (that is, before old age) of illness. This is similar to the situation with death from violence in the United States today—we are very aware of its presence. With medical progress, patients have come to believe that if there is an unanticipated result, someone is to blame and that death from illness should not occur. The medical profession has inadvertently fostered these impressions. The result is that managed care is tentatively pursued by health maintenance organizations. The organizations try to maintain patients' health while the patients do little to contribute positively to their health maintenance. The implication many perceive from a health maintenance organization is that if a patient joins the organization, health care be maintained regardless of initial health status or what the patient does. This is obviously unrealistic.

The idea that medicine can perform miracles has become pervasive because patients would like to feel they will live forever in a healthy state. On the clinical side, doctors do not want to dwell on failure. The downside is that patients do not have realistic expectations and health care providers do not correct the expectations very satisfactorily. Consider, for example, the situation in which a patient needs an operation. The surgeon suggests the procedure. The patient feels success is assured. Success is highly likely, but there can be unanticipated results. What should be done? To be told that death may result from the operation is not the best preparation for the patient, and, yet, death is almost always a possibility on a medically invasive procedure. It is generally true that, with respect to most operations, the most dangerous thing the patient does the day of surgery is to drive to the hospital. Both the patient and the doctor feel that success is highly likely, but neither may have true perspective: Medical care is usually choosing the better or best of several bad alternatives. The best alternative would be that the patient was not sick. A true perspective surfaces when the patient realizes that there are only alternatives, and some are better than others. The best choice is often based on what the patient needs with respect to living. Is it better to put up with gallbladder attacks or to have an operation that will almost certainly solve the problem, but carries a significant increase in short-term risk?

If the health care system could alter patients' perspectives about their own mortality, then risks and results of treatments could be considered without either assuming that everything will be fine, or effectively telling the patient that due to the serious operation, he or she may die. Helping patients to have accurate knowledge and perspective about their health has been brought into focus by legal liability and malpractice actions. It is important for these reasons and for cost considerations that patients be fully informed. In the final analysis, the imperative to inform is most crucial for moral and ethical reasons. Patients should understand and be able to make informed decisions even if it is difficult.

Implications of a Personal Contract for Care

This concept of the informed patient and a patient contract has serious implications in health care and distinctive benefits for care delivery, as shown in Figure 4.5. If individuals expect too much and the expectations do not come to pass, they are unduly upset. Unmet expectations may be the initiating factor in a great deal of legal liability—the patient expected perfect results in a situation in which perfect results were not possible. Realistic expectations could reduce legal liability as well as the cost of health care.

A formal contract, either accepted or rejected, might also change behavior. It is quite clear that patients would like to do some things with respect to health preservation. Even though informed, they do not seem to follow through on their responsibilities for maintaining health. A contract might help. Consider the case of pregnancies. Pregnancy is a perfect example in which expectations are often unrealistic. Pregnancy is safe, and desired results for mother and baby are almost always achieved. However, some studies have shown that when a woman becomes pregnant, her chances of dying within the next 12 months are increased by a factor of 10. Granted, the risk of death is very small and the rewards of a successful pregnancy are enormous, providing the baby is wanted. Nonetheless, in almost all other situations, human beings would think carefully about choosing one of two paths wherein their mortality is increased by a factor of 10. The result is that most women consider pregnancy without any regard to changes and most health care providers are totally optimistic about perfect results. The entire provider-patient interaction leaves the strong impression that results will be perfect. When-less-than perfect results occur, there is consternation. Realistic background knowledge would convey that becoming pregnant is a serious matter; it is quite safe, but it is certainly more risky than not being pregnant. All providers will do their best to ensure a good outcome for both mother and baby, but no guarantees can be made.

To achieve a realistic intervention between providers and patients will require a number of important changes. The concept of expert teams will help. However, managed care providers must also alter their approaches to marketing and promotion. Instead of implying that they are unequivocally the best, managed health plans must move toward defining their product, describing the ways in which they prevent rationing, how they reduce costs, and what they expect of patients. This comprehensive approach may seem absurd from a promotion and marketing viewpoint, but malpractice and legal liability are becoming so serious that no one who expects to remain in the health care business would consciously want to enroll anyone under the slightest false pretense. It may be better not to have any patients than to imply that you can do more than you can deliver. Thus, the intelligent marketing program would define the product or service, have clear boundaries, never promise what cannot be delivered and, ideally, deliver more than promised.

A personal contract for each patient is crucial upon entry into the system. The health of each patient should be evaluated in depth and discussed with the patient by a case manager. There is enormous difference between a patient who is healthy and one who is three-quarters dead. Too often today, all patients are considered the same regardless of health, exercise or ability to promote their own health. Then, once in the system, if patients have a heart attack or another serious health episode, each illness would be considered differently. It would be far better to assess each patient individually upon entry rather than imply that most heart attacks are similar.

With appropriate discussion, patients should better understand what options the providers recommend, what actions the patient should take in response, and what the patient can and will do. The patient's inability to do what is best should not be glossed over or changed by coercion. This contract will alter the legal liability and, in the future, might ultimately alter the price paid for the health care. Should someone aged 50 who smokes more than 50 cigarettes a day pay the same for health care as someone who does not smoke at all? If there is ever a differential cost, it should be with respect to actions the patient has some control over and not merely with the current health status that is involuntary. A price differential with regard to voluntary actions might help patients to alter behavior in a health-promoting direction.

REARTICULATION OF SERVICE DELIVERY

Medical facilities have evolved as a result of many changes and progress in medicine. Figure 4.6 illustrates this complex evolution. At first, contact between doctors and patients was either at the patient's home or wherever doctors practiced their profession. Scientifically, there was not much that could be done for patients until the 1900s. What doctors could do beside caring and exercising sound judgment could be easily carried with them in a bag. Serious care was delivered at home with a house call while office visits were made for follow-up or for maladies that were less serious. The value of patients coming to the office made doctors more efficient in a productivity sense. More patients could be seen in a given amount of time compared to making house calls.

Over time, hospitals developed as places to centrally care for patients. Resources could be concentrated so that better care was provided for very sick patients. As medical science developed, physicians discovered that many new operations could be performed more safely in hospitals. There were several trained individuals present if assistance was

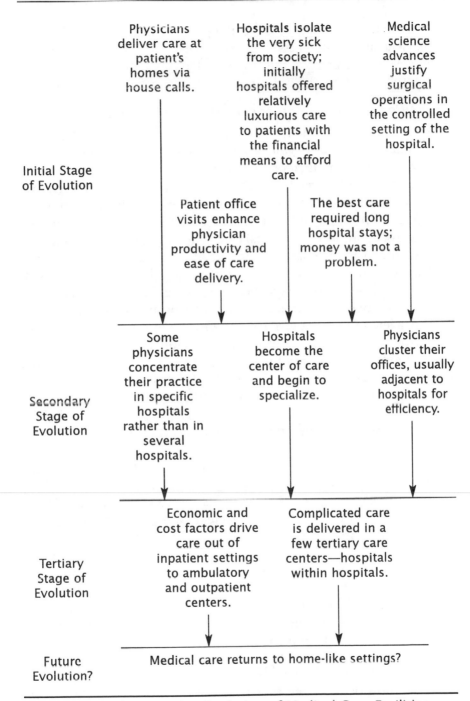

FIGURE 4.6   The Complex Evolution of Medical Care Facilities

needed. Some operations required the presence of more than one surgeon. General anesthesia could be more safely provided in a hospital. If an emergency occurred during an operation, the patient might survive in a hospital whereas she or he would not have survived at home.

Transition to the Contemporary Hospital/Medical Center

Over the past half-century, hospitals became the center of the health care industry. Doctors began to cluster their offices in buildings adjacent to hospitals for efficiency. Some physicians began to use one hospital rather than several. This was easier and more efficient for doctors, but enabled hospitals to compete with each other in a way that had not been possible before. These trends represent the secondary stage of evolution for medical care facilitators shown in Figure 4.6.

Because insurance paid for the care of patients within the system, and those without insurance did not receive equivalent care, new trends developed that made providing care easier for physicians. Many minor operations that had previously been completed in offices were delivered in outpatient operating rooms of hospitals. Where the minor operation was performed made little difference to the patient. For example, it was easier for a gynecologist to do a dilatation and curettage in the hospital. Theoretically, it was safer to have an anesthesiologist provide sedation in the operating room than for the gynecologist's nurse to give a shot in the office. Hospitals were delighted with the new trend. The only downside was that it might add more than $1,000 to a 10-minute procedure.

Another important trend occurred over the last half-century that represents the tertiary stage of evolution shown in Figure 4.6. Very complicated care for seriously ill patients developed as a result of medical progress. Furthermore, there were new heart operations, total joint replacements and advancements in infant delivery. For example, the time of viability for newborns has been pushed back almost 10 weeks. This progress made hospitals mandatory and, in effect, created hospitals within hospitals. Places such as intensive care units, newborn intensive care nurseries, burn units and other specialized centers developed to the extent that today, the term "hospital" does not really mean much in a descriptive sense.

The Future for Hospitals/Medical Centers

The evolution of complete care created a cost crisis. But, there is no single agreement regarding what is necessary in order to address the problem of uncontrolled costs. To make it more complex, what is necessary from the patient's point of view and what is necessary from the provider's point of view are often two conflicting ideas. Thus, we need to look at facilities as they exist and are used, and at medical requirements from several viewpoints (Wilson, 1998). Then we can consider what types of facilities would best fit the needs of everyone. Only at that point can we really determine how current facilities might be best utilized or changed.

Today, there are primarily three types of facilities in the main health care system: hospitals, physicians' offices and patients' homes. A patient's home is important because as hospitals have become excessively expensive, patients are sent home earlier and care is provided by visiting nurses. **Unless hospital costs are controlled, home care will become more important in the future.** Consider the problematic constraints that hospitals present. They are complex and expensive to build. They are not constructed in a way that makes them flexible. To enlarge the emergency department and reduce the size of an adjacent clinic usually requires extensive remodeling. There is usually a mixture of complex, noncomplex, and custodial care in a typical hospital. Food is expensive and often of modest quality. Personnel are seldom efficiently utilized—nurses trained in complex care may be providing custodial care for inpatients. From a cost point of view this is absurd. At urban hospitals and medical centers, parking is a problem and too often the surrounding neighborhoods are deteriorating.

There are also problems with physicians' offices. In urban areas, they are near hospitals so there are parking and crime problems. The location is good for the doctor and bad for the patient. Land is expensive so offices are expensive. There is a huge, fixed expense associated with buildings. If the neighborhood deteriorates, the hospital cannot be moved. Yet, the hospital by itself is not able to preserve a neighborhood. In most cases, offices are not equipped to do any minor surgery and certainly not to do most minor surgery.

Home care presents other problems. Increasingly, patients are sent home earlier. This is based on the fact that in a strict sense, hospital care is not required. Years ago, the hospital length of stay was much longer than necessary and now it is often too short—another reaction. For example, some insurance carriers used to pay for 24 hours in the hospital for obstetric care. If there are no complications with the birth, this is adequate for the mother, providing it is the first child and she has help at home. It is not adequate for her if she has other children (even if there is help) because the children will demand some of her attention and she will become more sleep deprived. In addition, the 24-hour rule may be strict, so that if the birth occurs in the evening, she will be discharged the next evening to start a night at home. This definitely is not good care. Mothers with newborns should be discharged in the morning and the choice should not be going home after 12 hours or going home at night.

The newborn as a patient is another matter. It is clinically questionable to send a newborn home in 24 hours and maintain certainty that there will be no problems. Consider the following experience. A very sick baby was diagnosed 40 hours after birth as having intracranial bleeding due to a congenital anomaly. The diagnosis was clear the second morning after an afternoon birth, but was not evident to experienced nurses in the newborn nursery at the time of the 24-hour discharge. The current system of early discharge overwhelms the patient too soon after having an operation. Theoretically, the patient does not need to be in a hospital from a medical point of view, but should not be discharged only to face all the attendant responsibilities. The necessary facilities to correct this problem are not available at the present time.

Toward a Sensible Solution

Figure 4.6 raises the question regarding whether the future evolution of medical care will observe a shift back to home-like settings (Parsons, Mahoney, & Weathers, 1999). It is crucial to consider what is required from both patients' and providers' points of view. Patients need to have correct facilities for medical and personal requirements. They require comfortable surroundings with some privacy when they are seriously ill (for example, those in intensive care units). Members of their family should be present with them 24 hours per day if patients desire. Patients deserve good food. And, patients should not be discharged until they are able to meet the responsibilities that they have at home. Such responsibilities may be different for each patient. Home implies an entirely unique set of demands.

We also need to consider the medical care needs that must be addressed if adequate facilities are to be created. Medical care requirements depend upon what is required for adequate care, not on the whims of a provider. These medical support requirements vary by diagnosis and they vary as an episode progresses. For example, patients who are severely ill with arteriosclerosis or other heart diseases and require personal care by experienced personnel (doctors, nurses, etc.). One patient may require the attention of several individuals (a cardiologist, an anesthesiologist, nurses). Then, after becoming stabilized, the patient will need one-to-one attention from an experienced nurse. If his or her condition improves, it is possible that in a short time one nurse can care for two or three patients.

This progression represents real changes in the patient's status and a reduction in the intensity of care. To be efficient, a reduction in care should be accompanied by a reduction in cost (not charges or reimbursement). Presently, hospitals are unable to effectively vary charges on the basis of acuity because they have not developed their accounting systems. A perfect example is found in postoperative recovery rooms. All postoperative patients are in this recovery room regardless of whether they have had a routine gallbladder operation or the most serious heart operation. Some are deathly ill and others are just waking up after a planned operation. Graded recovery units are not available and, thus, many patients had more care and the excess reserve of more care than they needed. Having this reserve instilled safety and was considered better quality. Such largess presented a limited problem until costs became important.

Some patient conditions are not immediately apparent with respect to diagnosis. Various signs and symptoms present for the patient elicit concern from the attending physician. But, the patient must be observed and have tests repeated over a 10-to-24 hour period. Formerly, these patients were admitted. Now there is pressure from insurance to send these patients home. This is dangerous and does not provide adequate medical care. Patients should be physically located where experienced personnel can make repeated observations as necessary. Also, personnel must be available if the patient's condition changes for the worse at any time. Do these patients need to be in a hospital? They are not necessarily sick now. They may not even be sick after observation. But, these patients should not be sent home.

In designing appropriate facilities to conform to medical requirements, a new model is desperately needed. There is evident justification for a residence-type facility that compromises the difference between hospital and home. To achieve this new setting will require a shift in thinking and the willingness to build a new paradigm of care. Hospitals were founded in order to promote a better system of medical care. Gradually, they forgot they were in the medical or health care business and thought of themselves as being in the hospital business. Some care must still be provided in the traditional hospital. There must be inpatient operating rooms, intensive care units (for example, general, newborn, cardiac, etc.) and burn units. There should also be step-down units for each of the intensive care units. Each of these functional areas should have well-defined standards and provide high-quality care. However, costs should also be controlled. To achieve this goal, as the units provide less-intensive care (that is, one-to-one nursing; then one-to-three nursing; then one-to-six nursing), the associated costs should decrease.

Step-down units could provide an intermediate area between the recovery room and the floor. It will be most effective if providers followed the diction to do what is necessary, but do not do what is unnecessary. As a result, hospitals could be designed more effectively. Most rooms in a hospital, including clinics, operating rooms and intensive care units, could be modular units that could be interchanged if requirements changed. This would help prevent institutional inertia that blocks flexible care delivery.

Instead of hospital beds, there should be residential facilities with hotel-sized rooms incorporating interconnecting doors so that a patient could be in one room and the family in the next. There should be hotel-type restaurants with room service and hotel prices. These services should probably be managed by a hotel. In fact, the entire residential facility should probably be contained within a hotel built adjacent to the hospital. The hospital would be reserved for acute care only.

A hospital could manage the residential facility except there would be a strong tendency to make the rooms more complicated and therefore expensive (that is, start with hotel rooms and subsequently design them into hospital rooms). The residential facility represents a setting where patients are getting better, not a place to be sick. Also, this facility should not be regulated by the groups that regulate hospitals (for example, JCAHO) or be subject to other hospital regulations required by the state. It is a hotel, not a hospital.

One nurse could be available for a given number of patients (for example, 1-to-10 or 1 to a floor). She or he will function like a visiting nurse and will make rounds twice a day. In addition, if a patient has a medical question or requests medical attention, the patient can call the nurse on the phone and arrange a room visit. If the patients are clustered for observation, the nurse might visit more frequently. It should be clear that this is not a hospital by another name. Patients are clustered for efficiency rather than being home. The nurse visits when necessary just like a home visit. The nurse is on call, not on duty in the usual nursing sense. At night, nurses would sleep unless called. This is a new concept that should have a cost of about one fifth that of a hospital room and, for many patients, would be better for their recuperation.

Residential care is different from home because patients are clustered and can be observed frequently over time. The patient does not have home responsibilities and yet can have access to family members. Medical personnel can easily see the patients as much as required for good care. Patients would be discharged from the residential facility when actually capable and confident of making the transition from supervised care to unsupervised living. This would probably be about the same time they were discharged from the hospital in the past. Between acute hospital and home, the residential facility represents an inexpensive place to stay that fits all medical and patient requirements.

Clearly, there will be many objections to this plan, as it requires health care providers to think in terms of a system rather than about their own vested interest. The health care system has lacked correct facilities for years. It has taken an obsessive emphasis on cost control to demonstrate just how obsolete facilities have become. At the very least, it will also take enormous innovation to properly reform the health system. As the residential facility demonstrates, patients, physicians and institutional providers (that is, hospitals) can anticipate a substantially innovative setting in which health care is delivered.

Electronic Relations

The current frontier in creating a patient-centered health care system centers on electronic relations. The Internet may be able to help patients access information and find care more readily in the future. Even at the present, a consumer can search the Internet to find valuable information on a particular condition. The primary problem is the varying quality of information. There is often quality information available for a disease or diagnosis, but finding that information can be very time consuming. There are no guarantees about the validity of the information once it is located. These problems are merely temporary and will fade away as health care providers realize that the

Internet can help them attract and retain patients while serving them more efficiently.

Wilkins (1999) has summarized the limitations of Internet access that currently make electronic relations problematic for health care providers. As shown in Table 4.4, consumers encounter at least five primary access problems. Some consumers are unable to pay for Internet service, which restricts their access from home. Related to this problem is the violation of employer resources by accessing the Internet at work. Consumers may also encounter considerable travel costs if they seek to access the Internet from a public venue. At the public venue, they may discover availability access problems in getting on-line. Once

TABLE 4.4   Access Issues and the Internet

Defining Access and the Internet		
Measure of Access	***Application to the Internet Definition for Health Care Stakeholders***	
Affordability	Ability to pay for services	Consumer does not have enough money to purchase a computer and cannot access the Internet from home.
Accessibility	Travel time, distance	Consumer does not have Internet access at home and must travel far to get access in a public location; particularly relevant for rural consumers.
Availability	Adequacy of supply in relation to need	There are not enough public and private Internet access locations to meet demand from consumers to get online.
Acceptability	Attitudes of consumers toward Internet	Consumers are afraid, do not understand how, or refuse to use a computer or an Internet Web browser.
Accommodation	Stakeholders do not meet consumer Internet constraints	Health care stakeholders do not accept accountability to enable consumers to get online and find valuable health-related information once they are online.

Source: A. S. Wilkins. (1999). Expanding Internet access for health care consumers. *Health Care Management Review, 24*(3), 30–41.

on the Internet, consumers may encounter access problems because of their dislike of technology or their lack of knowledge on using the technology. Finally, Wilkins notes that health care providers do not accommodate Internet access due to accountability issues.

Assuming that the access problems can be overcome, there are many reasons for health care providers such as physicians and medical groups to go electronic in their patient relations. Foremost, many patients want to know more about their illness and diagnoses. Those who are conversant with the Internet are especially drawn to providers who offer intelligent Web sites with medical information. Electronic relations may help to reduce administrative and clinical costs under some conditions. For example, if there is an influenza outbreak, a managed care plan may establish a chat room that is staffed by nurse practitioners. They can respond to questions (with the appropriate disclaimers) and educate patients. This may prevent utilization and could significantly raise patient satisfaction due to the immediate access to the managed care provider.

Wilkins (1999) has suggested that a number of Internet strategies are available to providers who want to expand Internet access, including the following:

- Provide community-based Internet access program;
- Provide "quality access" locations;
- Utilize telemedicine;
- Place computers/kiosks in public health care locations (hospitals, outpatient centers, clinics);
- Place computers/kiosks in public nonhealth care locations (libraries, schools, shopping malls, churches, synagogues);
- Place computers/kiosks in physician offices;
- Develop or direct consumers to educational programs on how to use computers, navigate the Internet and find health information on the Internet;
- Incorporate Internet consumer education into organizational and information technology strategic plans;
- Use clinical staff as online coaches to interact with consumers through chat rooms, e-mail or newsgroups;
- Use emerging, consumer-friendly technology (voice recognition, touch screens) to access the Internet;

- Direct consumers to Internet access locations;
- Target patients with chronic diseases in Internet educational efforts. Utilize software that enables sharing of information between patients and providers over the Internet; and
- Market the Internet as a health education tool.

In this view, these strategies can be considered by hospitals and health system and, to a lesser extent, by physicians and employers.

For physicians and medical groups the potential of electronic relations is impressive. However, in the short term, the primary problems in adopting one or more of these strategies will be initial funding. Electronic relations must make fiscal and care delivery sense. The best course of action is to develop a plan for using the Internet to meet patient needs. The plan should clarify exactly how investment in the Internet will decrease cost either through higher provider productivity or substitution for more expensive services. The plan should also consider the economic benefits from more satisfied patients and the drawing power of a sophisticated care system that upholds the finest patient relations.

APPLICATIONS FOR MANAGERS

In the last two decades, health care organizations have made considerable progress in the area of client and customer relations. Whereas once patients were treated as if they were lucky to receive services from physicians, there now exists a conscientious effort to build long-term relations. Unfortunately, payment mechanisms in health care often get in the way of forging such alliances. Many consumers are at the mercy of their employers when it comes to insurance coverage. Not every patient is able to remain with a provider or health plan year after year. This implies that medical groups and clinics have to work that much harder in cementing strong relations with their clients in providing the incentive for them to negotiate the insurance quagmire.

As this chapter has shown, a number of tools are available for medical groups interested in creating desirable relations with patients and clients. Perhaps the leading managerial approach involves assessing and monitoring performance of service delivery and client feedback. A wide variety of qualitative and quantitative methods are available from which to choose. However, it is important to recognize that no single approach is best. Instead, creating methodical and comprehensive assessment and monitoring methods offers the best promise for understanding how patients perceive a medical group's care delivery efforts. The key is to evaluate a wide range of performance areas while maintaining continuity in the assessment effort. This enables a medical group to identify areas of weakness and to purposefully design solutions.

It is easy to overlook the fact that assessment can be completed at a relatively low cost and, yet, significant benefits can be reaped for the effort. Most of the qualitative methods—management observation, employee feedback, quality circles and focus groups—do not require much in the way of resource investments beside staff time. The same is true for several of the quantitative approaches—comment cards, mystery shoppers and interviews. Surveys may require additional expense if the skills needed are not available internally. It is important to remember that the cost of undertaking customer relations assessment is miniscule compared to the returns on the investment.

Patient relations can also be managed effectively through benchmarking. Having collected basic information on clinic performance and client perceptions, medical groups can compare their report card to that of comparable providers. To the greatest extent possible, it is preferable to obtain indicators of performance from large numbers of similar organizations. Unfortunately, these data are not always readily available. However, this should not be an excuse for avoiding performance assessment. At the very least, medical groups can establish continuous monitoring of leading performance indicators as a way to benchmark performance.

A patient-centered care delivery model may use innovation to build relationships. Managed care plans and medical groups might consider personal contracts with patients as a means to involve them as active participants in the care process. A medical group does not have to be focused solely on managed care in order to implement this concept. It is conceivable that the majority of care delivery can include specific expectations for patients. This implies that patients will act as full partners in their own health care process. They will have better understanding of the diagnostic and treatment regimens. They will develop more realistic expectations of outcomes, and they will be better disposed to act appropriately relative to the intervention or management of their case.

Another step in creativity for managing patient relations involves rearticulating facility design for patient care. At the least-intense level, this implies restructuring how patients receive specific services—how services are bundled together, how patients enter a clinic and are physically processed, or how a group of clinics determines which specialties and subspecialties will be allocated among their ranks. For many medical groups in a single facility that has limited flexibility for alterations or for which excessive capital would be required to institute major modifications, the easy answer has always been do nothing but maintain the status quo. The times and pressures in health care make such an attitude a prerequisite for potential failure. Continuous improvement of patient relations suggests that medical groups examine every aspect of service delivery to ascertain innovative ways of serving patients better.

Medical groups that think they may have reached the point where they cannot possibly innovate further in terms of patient relations now are recognizing that electronic technologies offer a possible promising channel for new efforts. Younger generations of patients are clearly more adapted to, comfortable with and ready to use electronic means of communication. There are many opportunities to plan now for a future that capitalizes on electronic technologies to build patient relations. Given the speed of transitions surrounding e-commerce and the Internet, management terms in medical groups should meet frequently to plan methods for using these technologies as patient relations supports.

REFERENCES

Annas, G. J. (1997, July 17). Patients' rights in managed care—exit, voice and choice. *New England Journal of Medicine, 337*(3), 210–215.

Another record year for dealmaking. (1996, December 23). *Modern Healthcare.* (30), 37.

Asher, G. (1997, March/April). Improving patient access. *MGM Journal, 66*–72.

Bailit, M. H. (1997, November/December). Ominous signs and portents: A purchaser's view of health care market trends. *Health Affairs, 16*(6), 85–88.

Bodenheimer T. & Sullivan K. (1998, April 2) How large employers are shopping the health care marketplace. *New England Journal of Medicine, 338*(14): 1003–7.

Bradley, B. E. (1997). Putting patients first helps business. *Health Affairs, 16*(6), 121–122.

Chesanow, N. (1998, February 23). How one group builds market leadership. *Medical Economics,* 84–104.

Corrigan, J. M. (1995). How do purchasers develop and use performance measures? *Medical Care, 33*(1), JS18-JS24, Supplement.

Davis, K., Collins, K. S., Schoen, C., & Morris, C. (1995, Summer). Choice matters: Enrollees' views of their health plan. *Health Affairs,* 99–112.

Ford, R. C., Bach, S. A., & Fottler, M. D. (1997). Methods of measuring patient satisfaction in health care organizations. *Health Care Management Review, 22*(2), 74–89.

Forrest, C. B. & Reid, R. J. (1997, November/December). Passing the baton: HMOs' influence on referral to specialty care. *Health Affairs, 16*(6), 157–162.

Grandinetti, D. (1996, November 25). Teaching patients to take care of themselves. *Medical Economics,* 83–92.

Havinghurst, C. C. (1997). 'Putting Patients First': Promise or smoke screen? *Health Affairs, 16*(6), 123–125.

Ingram, B. L., & Chung, R. S. (1997). Client satisfaction data and quality improvement planning in managed mental health care organizations. *Health Care Management Review, 22*(3), 40–52.

Jensen, J. (1996, October 7). HMO satisfaction slipping. *Modern Healthcare, 26*(41), 86–88.

Kleinke, J. D. (1998, February 23). Power to the patient. *Modern Healthcare, 28*(8), 66.

Lee, P. V. (1997). The true test of whether health plans put patients first. *Health Affairs, 16*(6), 129–132.

Light, D. W. (1996). Primary managed care: More choice, less cost. *Medical Care, 34*(9), 985–986.

Mechanic, D., & Schlesinger, M. (1996, June 5). The impact of managed care on patients' trust in medical care and their physicians. *New England Journal of Medicine, 275*(21), 1693–1697.

Micheletti, J. A. & Shala, T. J. (1995). Case management can reduce costs and protect revenues. *Healthcare Financial Management, 49*(4), 64–70.

Parsons, M. T., Mahoney, C., & Weathers, L. S. (1999). Family suite: An innovative method to provide inexpensive postpartum care. *Health Care Management Review, 24*(4), 65–69.

Shortell, S. M., Gillies, R. R., & Anderson, D. A. (1994, Winter). The new world of managed care: Creating organized delivery systems. *Health Affairs,* 46–64.

Singleton, R. W. & Kilburn, N. (1995, November/December). Adding a mid-level provider to a group practice. *MGM Journal,* 30–48.

Tudor, C. G., Riley, G., & Ingber, M. (1998, March/April). Satisfaction with care: Do Medicare HMOs make a difference? *Health Affairs, 17*(2), 165–176.

Wilensky, G. (1995, Summer). Some thoughts on choice and satisfaction. *Health Affairs,* 78.

Wilkins, A. S. (1999). Expanding Internet access for health care consumers. *Health Care Management Review, 24*(3), 30–41.

Wilson, M. J. (1998, April). Enhancing managed care opportunities of group practices. *Healthcare Financial Management,* 58–61.

Yarmolinsky, A. (1995, March 2). Supporting the patient. *New England Journal of Medicine, 332*(9), 602–603.

Chapter 5

A Financially Viable
System of Care

Executive Summary

The sheer burden of rising health costs has driven the health care system to the point that change is inevitable or the entire system faces catastrophe. This is the backdrop to the role that medical groups play in creating a financially viable system of care. Despite managed care policies that have slowed the actual increase of costs in the health system, there remains an irreducible base cost of care—a level of costs that must be incurred in order for minimal quality of care to be delivered. Now, at the end of the managed care experiment, there is no other choice but to reinvent health services delivery. **Given the choice of reducing quality, rationing care, excluding care, or increasing productivity, it is clear that providers really only have one option—increasing the productivity of existing resources.**

This chapter examines team-based, patient-centered, procedural, facility-based and personnel strategies for enhancing productivity. Medical groups should consider all of these strategies when contemplating ways in which to achieve greater return on invested resources. The problem that most medical groups must overcome is the inertia of the status quo—the way things have always been done. Any of the productivity enhancement strategies require a willingness on the part of providers to reengineer the structure and process of care delivery. For example, a medical group might capitalize on nurse practitioners as a tactic to make triage more efficient. However, if the medical staff resists any deviation in the traditional process of care, it is unlikely that productivity gains will result.

Medical groups may have greater success at implementing productivity enhancements by instilling a metaphor of manufacturing within programs that restructures or reengineers care delivery. Medical manufacturing is comprised of three parts—the central concept and allied subelements of goal-oriented operating improvements; the infrastructure needed to implement the methodologies; and supportive programmatic strategies such as zero defects, functional specialization and goal-focused groups or teams.

COSTS AS A DRIVING FORCE FOR CHANGE

The United States has one of the best health care systems in the world at the present. There is, however, a significant exception that tarnishes its shining reputation. Health care simply costs too much. As a result, millions of patients do not receive adequate care. For them, the U.S. health delivery system is one of the worst systems in the world. From an economic viewpoint, health costs must be reduced. If many individuals do receive the right care at the right time with kindness, they certainly do not necessarily receive this care at effective cost. In reality, many receive care at the highest cost and others receive no care because they are not covered by insurance and have no money to pay for care.

Although managed care has contributed substantially toward lowering the rate of cost inflation within the health care field (Zwanziger & Melnick, 1996), a critical diagnosis suggests that it is not the envisioned solution (Johnson, 1995). Much of the escalating cost of health care arises from an attempt to patch together a system that is nonfunctional and fundamentally antiquated. An entirely new health care system must be reengineered.

EVOLUTION OF THE COST CRISIS

Within the last decade, there is increasing evidence that the price of health care must be reduced dramatically. Currently, the cost of health care delivery in this country approximates $1 trillion. It is estimated that $500 billion (that is, one-half of current total expenditures) must be saved in the next decade in order to preserve both the national budget and the integrity of the health care delivery system. Cost savings are presently being achieved, but mostly in ways that could destroy the entire system. Significant cost reduction is possible, but it will have to be achieved in very specific ways that do not destroy the entire system. Unfortunately, the most popular strategies for reducing costs based on controlling federal expenditures and capitating care delivery will undermine the system. Enlightened cost control must address other inputs in the service delivery process beyond revenues or reimbursement (Greene, 1996). However, solutions that would save the system are quite foreign to most health care providers, insurance companies, physicians, administrators, nurses and even patients. Some history is crucial in understanding the current dilemma.

The health care cost crisis has been evolving over the past half-century, as shown in Figure 5.1. In the early part of the 1900s, medical or health care was fundamentally in an embryonic stage from a financial viewpoint because there were no standard fees for doctors. Each physician decided his or her own fee schedule (Dixon & Trenchard, 1996). Some physicians charged all patients the same fee for the same treatment whereas others had a sliding scale of fees and

Time	Causal Factors for the Crisis
	Medical Profession Determines Payment Policies
Early 1900s	▪ Physicians set their own fees.
	▪ Physicians charge patients according to what patients can pay.
	▪ Physicians perform charity care as a noble professional act.
	▪ Physicians use more art (judgment) in care delivery than science.

Medical Profession and Third-Party Insurers Determine Payment Policies

Time	
Mid 1900s	▪ The fee-for-service method is introduced.
	▪ A specific fee is charged for a given service.
	▪ Higher fees are charged for specialists.
	▪ More referral and testing are undertaken to avoid litigation.
	▪ Charity care is eschewed.

Managed Care Plans Determine Payment Policies

Time	
Late 1900s	▪ Payers demand cost reductions.
	▪ Capitation is established and generalized.
	▪ Fee-for-service is minimized.
	▪ Care is contracted.

Lead to

Questions about the Best Cost-Reduction Strategies

FIGURE 5.1   Evolution of the Cost Crisis

charged patients according to what patients could pay. Almost all physicians performed some charity work and received no fee for this service. Providers practiced within a context of limited legal liability and minimal requirements for malpractice insurance.

Some order had to be imposed on the various service charges to avoid the wide variations surfacing among providers. As a consequence, fee-for-service care was adopted; that is, a specific fee would be charged for a specific service. This reimbursement approach seemed sensible and fair. Institutionalized, it would end the sliding scale fees used by some physicians to charge the rich more for care than the poor. Moreover, if a patient had health insurance or some third party to pay for care, fee-for-service reimbursement would make the entire process more consistent as third-party payers initiated oversight on physician charges and reimbursement.

Unintended Consequences from Payment/Reimbursement Policies

The fee-for-service concept created several unintended consequences and produced an enormously expensive health care system. There were several reasons, as suggested in Figure 5.1:

- A specific fee was paid for a given service. However, the fee was higher if a specialist performed the service. This encouraged the use of specialty care.

- The physician determining what service was necessary was the same one who received the fee. Physicians would receive more fees if they decided to perform more services. This did not mean that doctors necessarily performed unnecessary services, but over a period of time this policy tended to increase the cost of services to patients with specific medical needs because more specialty care was delivered. Patients and physicians assumed that more-intensive and expensive care was better than less-intensive and less-costly care.

- Legal liability became a driving factor in medicine. To avoid legal liability, physicians sought to remove ambiguity about their diagnoses and treatment decisions by extensive testing and referral. Producing the best medicine and the safest medicine resulted in more complex care but, potentially, care that had less risk for malpractice litigation. The end result was expensive care delivery.

- Over the years, health care institutions sought to avoid charity care. A prevailing view suggested that a fee should be paid for a service regardless of the type of patient. Furthermore, to many physicians, charity care appeared to be less than the best care, and physicians generally did not want to be associated with substandard care.

In effect, the fee-for-service concept dramatically changed the way medicine was practiced.

The Role of Payors in the Cost Spiral

Now, half a century later, the cost of care (particularly Medicare and Medicaid) has become an enormous problem (Gold, 1997). Employers and other payors are demanding that costs be reduced. Doctors are receiving guidelines from managed care plans on reducing costs. However, the problem is that no one knows exactly how to accomplish this elusive goal. Payors are putting pressure on providers in several ways, as suggested in Figure 5.1 (Conrad et al., 1998). One example of payor-induced pressure is capitation, wherein providers deliver total care (including care for complications) at a set price. There is limited ability to escalate price regardless of risk associated with complications or other factors that may increase cost to the provider. Another example of payor pressure for cost reduction occurs in negotiating decreases in fees for hospital services. This is a fundamental strategy by which health maintenance organizations (HMOs) reduce costs (Kertesz, 1998). For example, an HMO may negotiate with hospitals in its area to receive discounts. Another strategy by payors to reduce costs is (in the case of an HMO) to have several hospitals and/or physician groups in an area bid for a contract and then choose the lowest bidder (Trauner & Chesnutt, 1996).

Even if third-party payors and managed care plans are able to negotiate significant cost reductions, there remains some question as to whether the long-term prospects for controlling health costs are actually enhanced (Washburn, 1995). Figure 5.2 provides a visual portrayal of the problem that besets the enormous health care budget. An irreducible, basic cost of service is postulated. This is the theoretically lowest cost of delivering health care services that can be attained while preserving true quality. In other words, the irreducible cost of care is the point at which quality care is rendered at the lowest possible cost. The objective of the health delivery system is to reach this

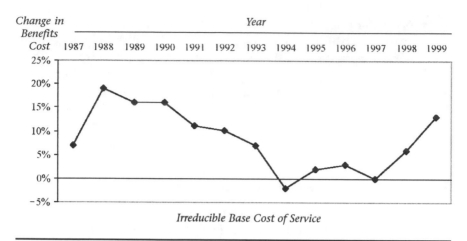

FIGURE 5.2 The Cost Spiral Dilemma

point but not to exceed it (Gamm, 1996). Below this line, inferior care is delivered at an inappropriately low cost.

The change in the cost of benefits—that is, the expenditures that actually occur in health delivery—is displayed as the varying horizontal line. The cost of benefits is depicted as rising precipitously until 1988, at which point it begins to decline gradually until 1994. Thereafter, the cost of service begins another gradual increase. A double-digit increase is predicted for the cost of health care services in the year 1998. In contrast, the irreducible basic cost of health care services is not projected to decrease.

In 1983, Medicare introduced prospective payment using diagnosis-related groups (DRGs). This was the initial signal to health care providers that things were about to change. Prospective payment essentially capped Medicare reimbursement for hospital services. Although the new policy had a modest impact on hospital costs, the far-reaching effects of revenue control soon became evident. The implications for additional reimbursement control by third-party payers were more vividly played out in ensuing years. In particular, managed care began to expand significantly in the late 1980s and early 1990s. Thus, in 1988, Figure 5.2 depicts a key threshold at which costs begin to fall more rapidly. Costs continued to decline until sometime in 1994. At that time, the negotiating capabilities of managed care plans were becoming marginalized as providers could not lower costs any further given the structure of their production (that is, service delivery) processes. Only very limited cost decreases were predicted after 1994, assuming that health care providers did not implement any significant changes in their delivery efforts.

There has been no appreciable erosion of the difference between the actual cost of service and the irreducible, basic cost of service (Iglehart, 1995). Here is the cost spiral dilemma in its most alarming form. Figure 5.1 implies that our efforts at controlling costs are little more than efforts at tinkering at the margins (Ryan & Clay, 1995). The health care system and health care policymakers are expending great effort with limited results. The tendency to continue down this path will only spell disaster in the end because the health care budget will remain a dysfunctional debt the nation must bear.

Cost-Reduction Strategies

As shown in Figure 5.3, there are essentially four ways to reduce costs: reduce overall quality, ration care, exclude payment for some unusual but necessary treatments or increase the productivity of the existing resources. Each medical group faces the same primary fiscal issues of how to reduce costs (Wood & Matthews, 1997) and how to reduce costs without adversely affecting quality or profit margins (Olden, 1996). Some explanation of what is meant by cost is in order. Traditionally, providers (that is, individuals and institutions) were paid a certain price for the services they provided (Cleverley, 1995). The price paid was based upon an agreed cost of care. This cost had been carefully negotiated by all involved and had been progressively determined over the years. The difference between price and cost was profit. This differential is being squeezed at the present time. Sometimes, the price paid is below the traditional cost. Hence, the precise strategy to adopt in reducing cost has become an important challenge.

Reduce Quality

There are numerous examples of reduced quality as a means for lowering costs. A typical approach in some groups is to pressure physicians to see too many patients per hour. If physicians have seen one patient every 15 minutes (four per hour), the group's administrative leadership may apply pressure for a new standard of six or even eight

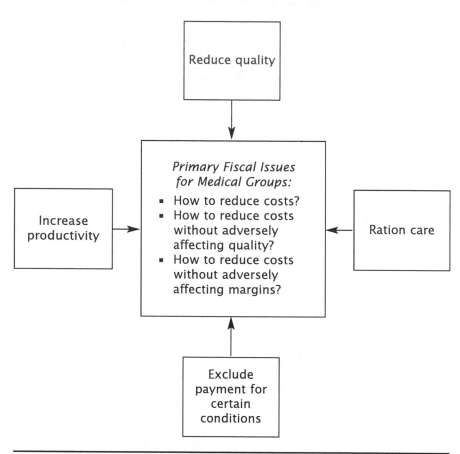

FIGURE 5.3   Cost-Reduction Strategies

patients per hour. Alternatively, physician remuneration may be reframed to achieve the same goal by benchmarking physician payment to the overall medical expense of the patient. The stipulated reimbursement assumes an average level of health status without adverse conditions. Thus, if a patient who is receiving care from a primary care physician has a heart attack, the reimbursement level could adversely affect the primary care physician's income. Another example of a cost-control strategy that essentially threatens to reduce the quality of care involves bonuses to physicians delivering patient care in a less-expensive manner. Physicians are potentially placed in an untenable position of taking shortcuts during care delivery.

Ration Care

The second way to reduce health care delivery cost is to ration care in a subtle manner. This cost-control approach takes two forms: first, indicated (but expensive) procedures are postponed as long as possible; and second, referrals to specialists are avoided. A patient may have the necessary symptoms and signs that would have provided an unambiguous indication for operation in the past. However, under rationing, the patient is encouraged (that is, forced) to wait longer to receive the operation.

A serious reduction in quality is occurring in medicine that is actually a combination of the first and second methods of reducing cost. Both quality reduction and rationing are employed. This situation involves general physicians who have difficulty in obtaining consultations from specialists or subspecialists. The history of family practice and the evolution of medicine provide numerous insights for understanding this phenomenon.

Family physicians, or general practitioners, evolved as a specialty in the 1930s. Prior to that, general practice physicians performed a wide range of services, depending upon their interests and skills. They performed surgery, obstetrics, gynecology and orthopedics. Then two changes occurred. Physicians specifically trained in some of the specialties—such as internal medicine, pediatrics, general surgery, obstetrics and gynecology, and orthopedics—achieved better results with patients for conditions related to their (sub)specialties. As a result, hospitals restricted doctors' admitting privileges in order to ensure the delivery of the best care. Consequently, general practitioners had difficulty in taking care of hospitalized patients.

This transition occurred because there was substantial new (and increasing) knowledge in medicine. One person could not know the latest clinical procedures and apply them compared to several individuals who only focused on narrower fields. Knowledge exploded in the past half century and this remains even more true in medicine today. If a knowledge explosion created the demise of general practitioners, then why is there a re-emergence of family practice in the last two decades? This phenomenon arose to solve another problem. As more specialists developed and some physicians became subspecialists, medical care became fragmented and serious problems developed with some patients. A patient might receive excellent heart care from a cardiologist and have a urological problem that was ignored.

Family problems were typically ignored by everyone. Serious illness of one family member generally affects others in the family. If two members had similar problems treated by different specialists, no physician necessarily had the knowledge of this occurrence or was able to look at the entire family. Thus, family practice emerged to solve this problem. There was one subtle caveat. A family physician could fully, without hesitation, call or send a patient to anyone more experienced if he or she felt that care would be improved.

One of the most serious and detrimental problems to achieving high-quality medical care occurs when a physician continues to care for a patient with problems the physician is not competent to solve. It is inculcated into medical students that they must know and freely accept their limits. Now, with the primary physician structure of most HMOs (that is, having a family physician, internist or pediatrician as primary care physician with real restrictions on the ability to consult or refer), primary physicians are essentially forced to do what medicine has tried to prevent for half a century. They must encroach on the turf of specialists. A reduction in care quality is inevitable. This is not meant to condemn family physicians, internists or pediatricians. There is too much knowledge, and one physician cannot do as well in most cases as several physician specialists who know more about the different problems.

The movement toward family practice in an HMO setting both purposefully and inadvertently rations care. Family practice purposefully rations care by instilling a gatekeeper who prevents patients from easy access to expensive specialists and subspecialists. It also inadvertently rations care because the family practitioner has more incentive to treat patients without involving the expensive specialist. It can be argued that patients will receive a lower quality of care because the family practitioner cannot possess as much knowledge in the specialized treatment of patients as the specialist for the appropriate condition. Although not every physician would agree with these assertions, it is clear that care rationing is more likely to result in the current health care environment in which such a premium is placed on controlling costs.

Exclude Payment for Certain Conditions

The third method of cost reduction involves excluding from payment necessary aspects of health care. For example, prescription medicine may be excluded even though it is necessary. Some new and expensive treatments for certain conditions may be discouraged or may be exempt from reimbursement. Unfortunately, scientific discoveries are being made that do make a difference in patient outcome, yet must be avoided due to excessive cost. For example, bone marrow transplants are being used in some treatments for cancer in conjunction with massive chemotherapy. In these cases, chemotherapy is increased to the point where it destroys the patient's bone marrow along with the residual cancer. Without the transplant, death would ensue quickly and with less massive doses of chemotherapy the chance of a cure might be less (for example, 35 versus 75 percent). Which option is best?

Increase Productivity

A fourth way to reduce costs is to increase provider productivity. The quality of care and the results for the patient would be the same under this strategy, but the real cost could be reduced. There are both fortunate and unfortunate aspects to this method. Fortunately, there is the possibility of reducing the true cost of health care enormously (probably as much as 50 percent) if this strategy is employed. Unfortunately, medicine is a profession with all the customs, guidelines and laws that stabilize a profession. To reduce cost and retain the same quality target would necessitate a shift in thinking with regard to how care is delivered.

PRODUCTIVITY AS A PROMISING STRATEGY FOR COST CONTROL

The promising solution for the cost spiral is to increase the productivity of all resources invested in health care delivery. This is why business concepts and practices could prove to be valuable in health care delivery. The history of medical care explains why so few efforts have been made to increase productivity. However, to modify productivity, physicians and medical groups must examine how services have been provided in the past and how the same (or more) services might be accomplished at reduced cost. Only a medical professional can complete this analysis and arrive at a solution that does not undermine care. So far, most of the cost pressure has come from nonphysicians—administrators, policymakers and managed care representatives—who contract to pay less or who put impediments in the path of expensive procedures or treatments. **If a satisfactory health care system is to survive, medical professionals (specifically the fundamental providers in medical groups, including doctors, nurses and support staff) must accept the cost challenge and think creatively about reengineering care delivery based on economics, quality, caring and accessibility rather than professional perquisites and professional authority.**

Productivity in the sense used here is the same definition as that used in business; that is, productivity equals the total cost of care for a group of patients over a period of time or the total cost of care for patients with a specific disease over a period of time. With increased productivity, total cost is reduced. This point is emphasized because, in medical terms, productivity has sometimes meant total charges of a physician over a period of time. The contemporary definition of productivity emphasizes reduction in cost while the traditional definition viewed by most physicians and medical groups emphasizes maximum charges. These concepts imply opposite business approaches and opposite medical meanings.

If costs are to be reduced and quality of care is to remain the same, medical professionals must utilize an exact process to reach the goal. Figure 5.4 depicts a process for productivity enhancement via reengineering in medical care (Ho, Chan, & Kidwell, 1999). The progression of steps in this process is crucial. First, the care provider team must decide what is the correct care for a patient with a certain condition. Then, the considerations of when to provide care are analyzed (that is, the right care at the right time). Physicians can accomplish both of these two tasks in consultation with technical specialists. The third and fourth steps must be decided by a cohesive group composed of providers involved in the care delivery process. If it is a medical clinic, then nurses, receptionists, and laboratory personnel may also join physicians in the process of setting care criteria. The third aspect involves determining how to provide care with the greatest kindness. The fourth step in the process is to consider a zero defects approach (six sigma). Care delivery should be implemented in a manner that avoids defects to the greatest extent possible.

After deciding what to do, when to do it, with the most kindness, and in a manner that produces the fewest defects, cost is considered. It is critical that the entire care team be involved for this step. The goal of the multifunctional team is to accept what has been previously

Productivity Enhancement Process in Medical Care Delivery

Step 1: Care provider team determines what is the correct care for patients with a given condition

Step 2: Care team decides the best time to provide clinical intervention

Step 3: Care team considers regimens for delivering care with the greatest kindness

Step 4: Entire care team examines process of delivery to ascertain how optimal end results can be achieved at reduced cost with no impact on quality

Facilitated by

Team-Based Strategies
- Cultivate a harmonious group
- Accentuate multispecialty values
- Reinforce group consensus

Patient-Centered Strategies
- Develop patient groups or cohorts requiring repetitive clinical services
- Create subspecialty groups for patients with consistent, unique conditions
- Reinforce group consensus

Procedural Strategies
- Reduce the complication factor in care delivery
- Balance short-term expediency against long-term benefits

Facility-Based Strategies
- Re-examine facility use assumptions vis-à-vis clinical severity
- Reconfigure services by facility to drive productivity of clinical teams

Personnel Strategies
- Alter care delivery to have physicians supervise less-expensive providers
- Redesign care delivery to substitute less-expensive providers for more/expensive providers

FIGURE 5.4 Strategies for Enhancing Productivity

decided (that is, necessary for quality) for care delivery and be creative in considering how the process can be completed with less expense and no deterioration in the quality of care, timing or degree of kindness. At this point, the group is operating expressly under the mandate not to change what has already been decided. When this specific approach is used, cost can be reduced without an adverse impact on quality.

This precise progression of events just described defines a methodology that recognizes important medical constraints as a first step. Cost issues are specifically reserved until the final step. Most efforts at cost reduction violate this process by considering costs along with what to do, when to do it and so forth. By considering cost reduction along with what care should be delivered, the focus tends to center on care delivery rather than on mechanisms for lowering cost.

Strategies for Increasing Productivity

Productivity can be increased if providers utilize ingenuity in clinical practice. In the past when cost was not a factor, there were many examples of inefficiency. Consider the case of a medical group with a busy surgical service employing three anesthesiologists and about 12 nurse anesthetists. The doctors supervised the nurses unless a patient was extremely ill. A new anesthesiologist became chairman of the group and within one year, there were 12 anesthesiologists and 12 nurse anesthetists for the same patient load. There was an enormous reduction in productivity.

Thus, there are often substantial variations in productivity, and there are numerous ways to increase productivity if creativity is used. The payment policies and ensuing cost problem generated by ill-conceived reimbursement strategies have removed the rewards and incentives to control costs. When third-party payors paid on the basis of cost, there was more money coming into the system if costs were high. Now, with capitation and negotiated contracts, there is no profit; and there is less funding for overhead and salaries unless the costs are low. Consequently, physicians and medical groups face a context wherein fresh thinking is needed to raise productivity in an effort to address decreasing revenue.

Another important factor to consider in strategies for enhancing cost control and productivity is patient shifting (Krentz, 1997). HMOs control enormous numbers of patients and can vary the providers who deliver care to specific patient cohorts. A medical group or hospital may have many patients one day and lose a substantial percent of its patient population to a lower-cost provider who successfully wins the contract bid. Moreover, with patient groups, there is the ability to organize care for the group in ways that were not possible when patients came in individually to receive care. Medical groups that participate in contract negotiations for managed care must fully recognize the advantage of caring for large patient cohorts; that is, the groups have an opportunity to exercise productivity enhancement strategies that are not available where small patient cohorts are involved. Thus, large patient populations possess a special value that can be utilized by medical groups (through productivity gains) in order to negotiate more competitively for managed care contracts.

Beyond the continuing search for opportunities to instill creativity in service delivery and the ability to reframe a medical group's perspective about the economic advantages of contracting for large patient populations, a number of productivity enhancing strategies are apparent, as shown in Figure 5.4. The productivity improvement process is the fundamental step (or series of steps) upon which additional strategies should be launched. Sidebar 5.1 provides an example of productivity enhancement in obstetrics that draws upon the strategies outlined in Figure 5.4. The process of productivity enhancement can be facilitated by team-based, patient-centered, procedural, facility-based and personnel strategies. Each of these will be examined in turn.

Team-Based Strategies

Several generalizations can be made about productivity. **One of the most successful concepts used to increase productivity in business is the multispecialty functional team.** In the practice of medicine, there have always been groups of individuals who have worked harmoniously together. For example, in a clinic there are doctors, nurses, receptionists and administrators forming the care delivery team. However, they have not always worked as a team in the sense that each subgroup had equal ability to make suggestions about how the provision of care was implemented. The same was true with automobile manufacturing in decades past. A car was designed, manufactured and sold, but these tasks were not necessarily coordinated by a team. Sometimes the car would not sell well in the marketplace because of the design or because it was expensive to manufacture due to the

Sidebar 5.1

Implementing Productivity Enhancement Strategies

Consider an obstetric service that must: (1) care for patients who enter the hospital in labor, (2) deliver babies and (3) assist mothers who are recovering after delivery. The obstetrics service will also encounter some pregnant patients who need to be hospitalized before delivery for obstetric or medical complications. Modern obstetric services must be able to perform cesarean sections on an emergency basis on the floor and care for these patients. Given these care requirements, several guidelines can be identified for productivity enhancement.

Guidelines for Enhancing Productivity	*Illustration in Obstetrics Services*
▪ Define standards for a minimum threshold of output, and determine number of providers available to deliver care	▪ Identify how many physicians and associated staff will provide care; identify how many patients need to receive care
▪ Establish an appropriate structure for care delivery	▪ Separate the care components (that is, patients in labor, patients in recovery, etc.); team members determine how care delivery will be organized

▪ Cultivate effective teamwork:
  ▪ Function is well-defined;
  ▪ Boundaries are set to prevent excessive change; and
  ▪ Stability is promoted
	▪ Specify the knowledge, experience, skills and attitude for each care component and match to team members' professional gifts/assets
	▪ Define and institutionalize the number of patients served per obstetrics team for a period of time
	▪ Have provider staff remain on a specific team and encourage them to resolve problems as a team; transfers are only seen as a last resort

▪ Inject creativity	▪ Assume that providers may substitute for each other; for example, technicians serving as scrub nurses, midwives serving as physicians in routine delivery
▪ Reinforce continuous improvement	▪ Have the team meet periodically to reassess the previous month's performance with an agreement that the meeting does not end until a distinct strategy for improving some component of service is adopted

continued

First, the standards for minimum service output must be defined:

- Are there only obstetric patients?
- What is the range of obstetric services that must be provided?
- How large is the service in terms of physicians, nurses and support staff?
- What are the constraints on space, personnel, money and associated resources?

When these parameters have been defined, the boundaries are established and not changed until the new plan has been implemented.

Different components should be considered with respect to personnel; that is, different provider skills are needed to address the different categories of patients:

- Sick, pregnant patients;
- Pregnant patients anticipated to deliver an uncomplicated birth;
- Labor patients, including monitoring;
- Patients during delivery and recovery;
- Postpartum patients after simple birth;
- Cesarean section patients; and
- Postpartum patients after cesarean section.

The provider team involved can decide who can perform various tasks most efficiently. What experience, knowledge and skills are required for each component? Are they cognitive or manual skills? What about breadth and depth of knowledge; are both required or is one more important than the other?

---

design. With a functional team approach, sales and manufacturing people have greater impact on design. In a similar sense, receptionists in a medical clinic have had very little say about the appointment or registration system. Few managers ever thought that receptionists might have suggestions about how to simplify the system if they were asked to make recommendations.

This was illustrated in a clinic at a university hospital in the Midwest. A registration and appointment system in the clinic required one hour for patients to complete necessary forms when they arrived and 40 minutes to complete necessary forms when they left. The entire process of serving patients was examined and it was discovered that all the necessary information could be obtained in 12 minutes when patients initially entered, and 4 minutes before they left. The old, antiquated system had just evolved over the years with providers adding information they felt was necessary.

If working groups are encouraged and required to function as true teams, a basis will be established for increasing productivity. **The multispecialty group that functions effectively as a team is the most basic element in increased productivity.**

Patient-Centered Strategies

Patient-centered strategies represent another approach that contributes to efficiency or promotes tactics resulting in greater efficiency. For example, similar patients can be grouped together to facilitate standardized processing. Subsequently, the groups can be separated to manage specific diagnosis and treatment regimens through more efficient methodologies. The groupings can be accomplished using several different criteria, such as problem severity, age or gender. Some patient visits are predictable and others are not. Some patients have serious problems that may take a long time and other visits are not serious. Some problems are emergencies and others are not. When different patients are appropriately grouped and appointments or visits are properly separated, staffing patterns can be adjusted for the maximum dysfunctional problem. Without the adjustments, there will be times when the providers cannot care for a specific patient in appropriate time.

The solution for effective grouping may be as simple as having a designated physician in the clinic see all urgent care patients who need an appointment that day. All the other providers can maintain their schedules without seeing emergency appointments. The diversity of urgent care problems and the variability in their severity can dampen productivity. However, the number of urgent care patients each day may be predictable, which means there can be planned staffing. The same approach is possible in the emergency department. There must be sufficient personnel with sufficient training to care for the worst situations that are unpredictable. Thus, by definition the urgent care and emergency care settings imply decreased efficiency in diagnosis and treatment, and consequently, in reduced productivity. Nonetheless, there is limited rationale for adversely affecting all providers' productivity. The medical group can plan for the highly variable cases while simultaneously gaining efficiencies from the less-variable cases.

If there is an adjoining urgent care center, the number of patients who are not serious (that is, they are able to wait 15 minutes) may be predicted as the clinic gains experience in implementing the patient cohort concept. The urgent care center can schedule appropriate staffing in view of these parameters and design the delivery process to care for most patients. The adjoining emergency department still must be maximally staffed for any possibility, but the extra staffing involves a relative minority of all staff needed to serve patients. This design is much less expensive.

Other strategies quickly surface. Using the batch concept in scheduling for a clinic or operating room and a unique ensemble of staffing has been helpful. Similar patients are scheduled together. It is far easier to have a continuous flow of patients. Consistent with a team approach, it is essential to receive ideas from all the providers involved on how to render the care delivery process more effectively. This batch approach instills operating efficiency that heretofore was less relevant in care delivery.

When doctors delivered care as solo practitioners, surgeons would usually operate one or more days per week and mix up major surgeries and minor surgeries in the course of their operating days. A gynecologist might do one major surgery and two different minor surgeries in a half day. However, it has been found that if they are busy enough to schedule similar cases, one after the other, greater quality and efficiency can be achieved. In most operating rooms, it takes almost an hour to do a minor procedure (for example, dilatation and curettage, sterilization, laparoscopy) when they are mixed up with major cases. Contrast this to a medical school hospital in which a department started diagnostic dilatation and curettage in the clinic under local anesthesia. It was discovered that one physician could do four dilatation and curettage procedures in one hour (for example, a four-fold increase in productivity). Today, with HMOs sending large numbers of patients to medical groups, the batch concept in scheduling must be utilized in order to achieve pertinent care delivery goals.

Procedural Strategies

In providing the best care with no restraints on cost, physicians have tended to make practice more complicated (and more expensive). Many examples illustrate this dysfunction. Patients may be discouraged from eating after an operation simply as a safeguard. In many postpartum situations, 90 percent of all patients could eat successfully after delivering their babies. Nonetheless, over the years surgeons and hospitals discovered that it is easier to wait than to feed everyone and worry that 10 percent will have problems. Unfortunately, few hospitals or physicians even consulted the patients for their preferences. Alternatively, patients may be given an intravenous (IV) solution so that medication can be injected into it. An IV costs more than $100 for a several-hour period. In contrast, a heparin or saline lock can often accomplish the same function at a cost of about $30. Medication, whether given intravenously or intramuscularly, involves a disposable syringe and needle. If the medication is given directly into the vein or muscle each time, the cost is only for the needle and syringe. A patient who is going to receive medication only one time will have the vein punctured in any event, but the cost may be for a syringe alone; syringe plus $30; or syringe plus several hundred dollars. In the past we have never considered this cost of what we do and how we do it.

Another aspect of procedural simplification involves treatment. For a given medical problem there may be a partial solution that temporarily relieves a condition and thereby avoids a more definitive solution (that is, possibly an operation). HMOs encourage physicians to pursue the incremental partial solutions because these temporary means often appear to be less expensive. However, they may not be less expensive when all of the steps are combined. Whether or not they are cost efficient depends upon the likelihood of success. If a patient has little chance of success, it is less expensive to move to the definitive solution immediately. In many cases, the patient would like to have this explained and participate as a partner in the choice.

The preceding examples convey that procedural strategies at productivity enhancement are designed to improve the process of care delivery (Bachman, 1997). In business applications, this approach is typically viewed as reengineering. Careful study is undertaken to identify opportunities in which improvements can be instilled (usually by all representatives of the parties involved in the production or service delivery process). Clinical applications have risen in recent years, but the quality improvement processes in health care usually violate the fundamental assumptions of redesign. Normally, in clinical situations, the quality improvement effort seeks to fine-tune an existing process or set of procedures. Seldom does the continuous quality improvement process begin at a zero base before reconstructing the clinical application. This inadvertently leaves dysfunctional elements in the service delivery process—elements that then require substantial maneuvering on the part of the care team in order to resolve the problem adequately.

Medical groups that are able to encourage bold or complete reconsideration of care process basics have a better opportunity to build relatively error-free regimens (Van Horn, Burns, & Wholey, 1997). The downside of such thorough reexamination is, of course, the time invested in reinventing the process. Granted, the short-term costs in staff time and effort may be intimidating. Busy physicians and other clinicians are usually focused on delivering care now rather than later. Nonetheless, the progressive medical group focuses on the long-term benefits from investments at improving service delivery processes.

Facility-Based Strategies

Appropriate facilities are another area that promises possible increases in productivity. However, the tendency on the part of providers to think traditionally often stymies improvements. For example, many patients enter the hospital for observation. To decide the medical status and most promising intervention, the patient must be followed closely by doctors and nurses for 24 hours. Providers cannot see patients every two hours if the patients are at home. Thus, patients are admitted for an extensive and very expensive inpatient visit. However, providers could observe a patient in an adjoining hotel at a fraction of the cost of the hospital. The same is true of postoperative or postpartum patients. As long as clinical procedures are not being performed, there is no economic or quality of care benefit from being in the hospital. Whether or not patients are sent home too early from their point of view is determined by the home situation (that is, is there someone to help them or do they have to immediately take full care of their family).

Facility-based strategies require substantial rethinking about care delivery from a nontraditional perspective. The challenge is to devise innovative or ingenious ways that do not reinforce the typical approaches, assumptions or applications prevailing in health care. It takes considerable courage to go against the grain in proposing radical alterations to service delivery. The status quo acts as an enormous constraint on the creative redesign of health delivery systems. Penetrating analysis inevitably will encourage clinicians to question the assumptions upon which they perceive the appropriate and necessary uses of health facilities. Once they view facilities as sites for care delivery rather than as institutions with a predetermined function, the possibilities for innovation soar and, along with this fresh environment, the possibilities for more productive use of the facilities.

Personnel Strategies

Finally, enormous increases in productivity can be made if people are used more effectively. There are three very important groups to consider: physicians, nurses, and midlevel providers such as nurse practitioners and nurse midwives who are licensed to perform certain medical tasks independently (Lowes, 1998). This is not to suggest that other critical support staff such as technicians and auxiliary support personnel cannot also be employed in an improved, substantive fashion. Nonetheless, the Pareto Principle applies in that 80 percent of the cost reduction in care can be derived from 20 percent of the vital care providers. Classically, physicians as experts have done the actual work of caring for patients themselves. In the future, it will be more efficient and may be necessary for physicians to supervise others for much of the actual care.

Personnel strategies for productivity enhancement typically center on techniques for making existing personnel more productive. Sidebar 5.2 provides one example of how staff can be made more productive. The legacy of global competition within the business sector clearly points to intensive efforts by corporations to squeeze out more production per worker because the highest costs of production are often labor costs. Businesses have attempted two key strategies to reconcile the high cost of labor. One approach has been automation that essentially replaces machines for personnel. However, this tactic is capital intensive. Unless production runs are extremely long (that is, decades as opposed to years), there is often a question as to whether the capital costs can be recovered. The rapid product obsolescence characterizing the global marketplace argues persuasively against optimism for long production runs without significant retooling. Product life has shortened dramatically and, hence, brings into question the wisdom of capital-intensive production equipment.

Another tactic employed by businesses to enhance productivity and profit margins is to seek the lowest-cost labor. Athletic shoe manufacturers have become notorious for building instantaneous production facilities in geographic areas where labor costs have not risen. Using portable machines/tools and simplified manufacturing processes, these firms keep their labor costs down by remaining agile. Once

SIDEBAR 5.2

Enhancing Productivity by Reassigning Tasks

In medical groups that are truly interested in productivity enhancement, traditional tasks are being examined to determine critically which staff member should perform specific tasks. In obstetrics and gynecology, the following evolution of task assignment is predicted:

Clinical Task	Traditional Provider	Current Provider*	Future Provider
▪ History taking	Physician	NP, PA, RN	Nurse
▪ Evaluation of lab work	Physician	NP, PA, RN	Computer
▪ Physical exam of normal patient	Physician	NP, PA	Nurse
▪ Preoperative screening	Physician	NP, PA	Nurse
▪ Postoperative care	Physician	NP, PA	Nurse
▪ Surgical assistance	Physician	PA	Nurse

*NP = nurse practitioner
 PA = physician assistant
 RN = registered nurse

The primary point is that the traditional health care delivery system has often relied on the least-efficient resource deployment to accomplish the task at hand. Physicians have traditionally been assigned tasks that others could complete in an effective manner if efficiently organized and managed. If the health delivery system is actually expected to attain optimal resource efficiency, significant alterations will be necessary, not only in who completes which task, but also in how tasks are configured.

the wage structure of a community begins to rise to the point that margins are threatened, the firms merely transport the production facilities to the next setting of low-wage rates.

For the most part, medical groups cannot emulate their business counterparts by replicating these popular personnel strategies for raising productivity. Health care providers cannot afford to constantly move operations because their patient populations remain fixed, and providers can only substitute a limited amount of technology to replace personnel. In the final analysis, the delivery of health care services still relies predominantly on people for rendering care. Admittedly, scientific advances in medical technology continue, but the outcome of these technological advances is primarily related to technical aspects of diagnosis or treatment—not productivity enhancement for providers. Furthermore, the technology that has improved provider productivity generally is centered around technicians. While raising the production of technicians is desirable, the high-cost labor for physician care remains relatively unaffected by new technology.

The most promising opportunities for productivity enhancement among the mainline clinicians—physicians, nurses, and mid-level providers—involves who actually delivers care (De Angelo, 1995). To this point, the medical community has insisted that physicians play a high-touch role in patient care. Responsibility for diagnosis and treatment remain the purview of physicians. This convention essentially dictates that care will be provided by the highest-cost labor. Consequently, the medical system is rapidly approaching a point where either physician wages must decrease (if they continue to play such a pervasive role in clinical care) or they must supervise care rather than deliver it directly. This suggestion is very troubling because physicians do not want to alter their authority or direct involvement in the care delivery process, nor do they wish to experience lower salaries. Moreover, physicians often overlook the indirect benefits that accrue from delegating care to others such as mid-level providers. Sidebar 5.3 captures many of these indirect benefits. However, if health care costs are to be reduced, one or both of these alterations will be necessary.

BARRIERS TO PRODUCTIVITY ENHANCEMENT

Several barriers or problems are emerging in health care with distinct ramifications for productivity. These barriers could constrain efforts at productivity enhancements and reengineering by medical groups (Arndt & Bigelow, 1998). One barrier involves the façade of physician extenders. For example, nurse midwives, nurse practitioners, or physician assistants may be hired under the guise of improving productivity when the real objective is to make physicians' lives easier. Midwives and other mid-level professionals will not necessarily be

SIDEBAR 5.3
Indirect Benefits from Using Mid-Level Practitioners

In a review of the potential value from using collaborative practice to lower costs and increase productivity, De Angelo (1995) observed that the Carle Clinic in Urbana, Ill., had progressively adopted mid-level providers to address patient access problems. De Angelo notes that physicians often were unaware of the indirect benefits surfacing from the use of mid-level providers; benefits that were enjoyed by the physicians themselves as well as patients and the Carle Clinic.

Indirect Benefits for Physicians:

- Continuity of care for absences or rotations;
- Enhanced patient education;
- Opportunity to care for more diagnostically challenging patients;
- Opportunity to see paying patients while NP/PA sees "no-charge" visits;
- Increased OR time for surgeon when initial rounds, pre- and postop visits are made by staff;
- Practice relief in single-specialty practices;
- Decreased need for additional primary care and specialist physicians; and
- An alternative for educational responsibilities with medical school.

Indirect Benefits for Patients:

- Access to care—less waiting time for appointments;
- Time for education/questions;
- Care continuity;
- Reduced health care costs; and
- No co-pays.

Indirect Benefits for the Carle Clinic:

- Public relations;
- Cost-effective resource for managed care population;
- A focus on prevention education;
- Increased compliance with treatment requirements;

continued

- Less costly providers for some services such as nursing home rounds;
- Access in locations where physician recruitment is not satisfactory;
- Additional resource for staff;
- Flexible primary care staff pool; and
- Resource as faculty for medical school, nursing school, community groups.

These indirect benefits were in addition to the dramatically increased revenue from higher patient services.

Source: Adapted from L. De Angelo, (1995, November/December). Collaborative practice. *MGM Journal*, 12–18, 85.

embraced by physicians in the care delivery system or by patients. From a cost point of view, they can perform many tasks routinely done by physicians; that is, nurses can function as true extenders rather than just assistants. Nurses can and have delivered far more patient care than meets the eye.

Sidebar 5.4 provides examples of how various medical groups have effectively used mid-level providers. If physicians open themselves to opportunities for mid-level personnel to enrich patient care, the implications for increased productivity are impressive. Again, an efficiency contribution alone does not guarantee that physicians, patients or providers will embrace a different care approach. Nonetheless, higher productivity that can lead to lower costs should provide an incentive to physicians and medical groups to reinvent professional practice relationships.

Another barrier to productivity to consider centers around the tendency of many doctors to retain tasks that others could just as well perform. Medical groups and physicians can perpetuate this mentality if they are not interested in lowering costs. Eventually someone will consider the prerequisites for the tasks and if a staff member can perform the tasks as well and at less expense, physicians' income (and health costs) will be reduced accordingly. **The emerging forces for cost control and productivity enhancement suggest that a service is worth as much as it costs to have someone do it appropriately with outstanding results.**

SIDEBAR 5.4

Successful Clinic Applications of Mid-level Providers

Whom do you choose—a nurse practitioner or a physician assistant?

Psychologists are midlevel providers. So are occupational therapists, nurse midwives, and social workers. But when most group practices think of hiring an MLP, they think of a physician assistant or nurse practitioner to help their harried primary-care doctors.

But which one? In terms of their capabilities, NPs and PAs are more alike than different. But you may gravitate to one or the other depending on your patient population, your doctors, and state laws defining MLPs' purview.

Physician assistants, whose specialty gained impetus from medics returning from the Vietnam War, generally train in two-year postgraduate programs. Most who work in primary care are generalists in the FP mold. In a typical day, PA Randall Ideker at Group Health Permanente in Lynnwood, Wash., for example, might treat someone with the flu, remove a toenail, splint and cast a simple fracture, counsel a depressed patient, and prescribe a painkiller for someone with a gall-bladder problem.

Nurse practitioners—RNs with advanced education and clinical training—tend not to perform as many procedures or see as many patients as PAs do. Instead, they're more likely to subspecialize in primary-care fields such as pediatrics. NPs place a greater emphasis on patient education, and, in general, reflect a nurse's concern for the whole patient. "Because of my training as a nurse, I don't consider just the physical problem at hand, but what's going on in the home," says pediatric NP Nancy Quigley at Health Key Beacon in St. Louis.

Groups with a track record of using midlevel providers say there's no dramatic difference between PAs and NPs. "I don't draw too many distinctions between them," says Greg Trerotola, CEO of Pentucket Medical Associates in Haverhill, Mass. However, Group Health Permanente hires more PAs than NPs in part because the latter belong to a union that has gone on strike several times in recent years, say GHP officials. The NPs' union status also bars them from becoming shareholders-a right enjoyed by PAs. The line between the two types of MLP is so thin that such factors can be decisive.

If anything, PAs pose less of a psychological threat to doctors, since their state licenses hinge on physician supervision. NPs, in contrast, are

continued

licensed independently, and can practice without physician collaboration or supervision in 25 states and the District of Columbia.

Practice management consultants advise groups to match MLPs to their patient population. "If you have a standard FP practice with a balance of young families and geriatric patients, you might want to go with a PA, because they're more well-rounded," says Dorothea Taylor, a consultant with The LaPenna Group in Kentwood, Mich. "But if you're a pediatrician or OB/GYN, NPs are a natural choice, given their specialized training. And since so many of them are women, they bond well to mothers and moms-to-be."

The choice eventually boils down to personal chemistry between a prospective MLP and a physician, says MLP administrator Thomas Robinson of the Ochsner Clinic in New Orleans.

"It's not an either/or with NPs and PAs," says Robinson. "You just need the MLP who's the best fit with the doctor."

Source: R. L. Lowes. (1998, April 13). Making midlevel providers click with your group. *Medical Economics*, 131.

A third barrier to productivity is excessive staffing. Overstaffing for situations that rarely occur is another people-related causal factor for low productivity. Medical groups should match appropriate staffing to the appropriate circumstances. Such a strategy promotes lean production in the whole organization; that is, a value stream in which more can be achieved with less.

A fourth barrier to productivity in health care that inhibits attaining effective cost is the personal attitude and behavior of patients. Often, patients do not understand enough about their health conditions to take personal responsibility for their care. When patients do have actual and emotional understanding, they are better able to form strong partnerships with providers to enhance their personal health care. The lack of understanding is based on several things: Some lack knowledge; some deny their health problems; others have emotional blockages resulting from the denial; and other patients possess a mentality that providers are servants. Without true actual and emotional understanding, patients cannot make the best decisions, cannot help themselves and cannot contribute to lower costs by helping providers improve their efficiency (and, hence, productivity) in delivery.

COST CONTROL THROUGH THE METAPHOR OF MANUFACTURING

Medical groups benefit substantially when their leaders step out of the box of traditional thinking to gain fresh perspectives on how services and staff are organized. Particularly in the health care delivery arena, there is notable value in examining business manufacturing and service efforts as a means to gain better understanding of alternative strategies for medical group operations (Preston, 1997). In many respects, the metaphor of manufacturing is very apropos to the medical group context. Although medical groups and physicians may be hesitant to acknowledge that they need a shift in resource productivity, it is clear that outside of raising revenues and controlling costs, the most promising strategy for improving health care delivery is in deriving greater productivity from resources used. We contend that substantial, real productivity gains are feasible in medical group settings if industrial manufacturing concepts are applied more liberally. However, it is unrealistic to believe that the metaphor of manufacturing will be easily embraced across the broad spectrum of health care providers due to ingrained attitudes about patients and the care delivery process. Nonetheless, there are compelling forces that inexorably encourage widespread adoption of manufacturing concepts.

Traditional Care Delivery Philosophies that Constrain Productivity

For more than half a century, productivity in medicine referred to the amount of money physicians charged in the course of delivering care; that is, the charges resulting from patient care. This charge-revenue relationship was viewed as optimal when total revenues (or charges) were at their highest. From an economic perspective, this was an unusual approach to defining productivity because it omits the concept of efficiency, or the output for a given level of input. Total charges actually represent the level of production—not the level of productivity. Medical productivity is now based on a more business-like (or economic) definition associating maximum service with minimum costs (rather than with maximum costs). This is a very difficult conceptual bridge for physicians to cross because they have tended to equate charges with costs.

New methods of reimbursing providers are focusing more attention on medical productivity due to the declining margins of capitated care. The goal in increasing productivity is to care for more patients with less cost. Certain modifications in care delivery can be made while using the same personnel (that is, a fixed work group) in order to enhance productivity. Anyone observing a health plan or clinic after a fixed-cost contract has been instituted will likely observe examples of these changes. Figure 5.5 depicts several strategies for altering productivity and the vacuum they create for more intelligent and innovative responses.

First, the same group of people can attempt to produce more during the same hours. As Figure 5.5 indicates, they typically will take fewer breaks, shorter lunch periods, and scramble more while they

---

Medical Group Responses to Capitated Care

Work Harder	*Work Longer Hours*	*Reduce Payment for the Same Work*
▪ Take fewer breaks; ▪ Take shorter breaks; ▪ Shorten lunch; ▪ Scramble more; and ▪ See patients for fewer minutes.	▪ Lengthen days; ▪ Shift administrative work to weekends; and ▪ Add clinical hours on the weekend.	▪ Decrease salaries; ▪ Terminate bonuses; ▪ Constrain pay increases; and ▪ Hold salaries level.

Create the
Need for

System
Modifications

- ▪ Innovative solutions in addressing productivity enhancement;
- ▪ Options that do not penalize providers;
- ▪ Solutions that do not sacrifice quality for the sake of cost; and
- ▪ Long-term thinking.

FIGURE 5.5   Ill-Fated Productivity Responses to Fixed-Cost Contracts

work. With respect to physicians, they can take less time with each patient and see more patients per hour. All of these changes reduce some of the fat in the system. These changes may or may not result in poor-quality care or more mistakes. The amount of heightened productivity attained depends upon the level of inefficiency and the reward for reducing it.

Another alternative for raising productivity shown in Figure 5.5 is to have the same personnel work longer hours so that they can take care of more patients. How upset the individual providers will be depends upon how many hours per week they were working before the shift. This productivity strategy has clear limitations due to human resource constraints.

A more upsetting alternative is to reduce payment for the same work. This can be achieved either by reducing or terminating bonuses (if there were any to begin with) or reducing salaries. Another way to reduce salaries is to avoid pay increases or pay a less-than-planned increase. Either of these two strategies can elicit substantial dysfunctional reactions from staff.

All three methods result in paying less for the same or more work. All three methods—working harder and faster, working longer hours, and reducing payments—are short-term solutions and tend to reduce the quality of care. How well they work in the short term depends upon how much inefficiency exists, how upset the providers become, and whether or not they agree that costs must be reduced. A better solution is to modify the system as suggested in Figure 5.5. The following example demonstrates that there can be true cost savings and no adverse reduction in quality, thereby achieving proper economic and productivity gains if innovation is added to the equation.

There was a severe shortage of latex for surgical gloves in 1988 because of a need to produce more condoms for autoimmune deficiency syndrome (AIDS) protection. The shortage became so severe that surgical operations were on the verge of being curtailed. Traditionally, for an operation like a dilatation and curettage, an operating room crew might use four pairs of expensive latex surgical gloves: one nurse would use one pair to set up the surgical room, another nurse would use a pair to prep the patient, the doctor would use a pair for the operation and a nurse would use a pair to clean up. They reduced this waste by having one nurse use one pair to set up and prep the patient. The doctor used one pair, and one pair of nonsterile, nonlatex gloves was used for clean-up. This resulted in a significant cost savings while making providers more productive because they were not constantly changing surgical gloves.

Contemporary Philosophies that Increase Productivity

Significant gains in productivity can often be made by having providers work differently or, as has become known in the literature on reengineering—working smarter (Yasin, Czuchry, Jennings, & York, 1999). This might sound easy, but in fact it is quite difficult because of the implication that individuals will not continue to function in the same, traditional way. Productivity gains can be effectively blocked because few people like to change. In fact, companies throughout most industrial sectors discover that efforts to increase productivity require an enormous amount of pressure. In many cases, a shift in thinking is essential to instilling change.

There are numerous, subtle examples of low productivity in medicine. The way in which most operating rooms function is illustrative. Traditionally, individual surgeons scheduled cases at random so that it was unusual if the same surgeon performed back-to-back operations to any great extent. As a result, one surgeon operated and then the room was used sporadically the remainder of the day. In an eight-hour operating period, as much time may be spent in changing patients as in actually undertaking the operations. In other words, there might be four or five hours of actual surgery and three to four hours of getting patients in and out of rooms. Most clinicians who have never seen another system will feel little can be done to improve productivity. However, a different reality exists. For example, a few years ago at a leading medical clinic, surgeons were provided the availability of two operating rooms on their day to perform surgery. It was found that the number of operations a surgeon could do was doubled by this method when there was no waiting to have the patient taken out, the room cleaned, and another patient brought in.

An extreme example of heightened medical productivity was described by an ophthalmologist in Pakistan. There were many patients with cataracts, and he was essentially the only eye surgeon in the country at the time. There were no screens on the windows or doors in the hospital and no heat or air conditioning. Hence, he could only operate when there were no flies and when the temperature was moderate. This turned out to be a two-month period during the year and only from about 4:00 a.m. to 8:00 a.m. each day. The physician rotated among several operating rooms. The only part of the operation he performed was the actual removal of the cataract. On a daily basis during this period, he operated on 200 patients per each four-hour period.

Toward the Concept of Medical Manufacturing

To achieve the preferred outcomes necessary for the survival of the health care delivery system—low cost, high quality, and high productivity—will be an enormous undertaking. How medical groups can deliver the results is a significant challenge. The term "medical manufacturing" is a useful metaphor for an efficient, business-like approach that medical groups should strive to accomplish.

There are three fundamental components underlying medical manufacturing. The first part defines the central concept and key elements of medical manufacturing. The second component concerns the infrastructure needed to implement the methodologies, and the third element describes supportive, programmatic care strategies. Together the components represent a powerful concept aspiring to deliver the right care, at the right time, at effective cost with kindness, as shown in Figure 5.6.

The Central Concept of Medical Manufacturing

The central concept of medical manufacturing shown in Figure 5.6 requires that a protocol be strictly followed so that for all patients with a given condition, tests for diagnosis and treatment are the same (Smith, Yourstone, Lorber, & Mann, 2001). The protocol must ensure that the right thing is done at the right time, at the right cost and with kindness. It should be clear that a cohesive system of care is necessary to reach this visionary goal. The essential concept implemented in any given medical clinic encourages a consistent and identical product for a given set of circumstances. For a specific set of signs and symptoms, all patients will have the same steps for diagnosis and will be treated in the same way. A protocol will be developed that incorporates the best thing for these patients, considering kindness and cost as measured by outcome. A team will develop the protocol with the idea of functioning as a cohesive unit rather than as a divergent group of individuals. Some patients will fall outside the protocol. They will be exceptions. However, the goal is to include patients in all

Central Concept of Medical Manufacturing

Care delivery protocols are carefully designed so that all patients with a given condition receive the same care management. Each protocol delivers the right care at the right cost with kindness and quality.

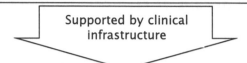

Supported by clinical infrastructure

Clinical Adaptations to Implement Medical Manufacturing:

- Protocols are developed to ensure a consistent and identical product/service for a given set of conditions.
- Protocols drive team cohesiveness by integrating team members in the creation, refinement, and assessment of care delivery processes.
- Patients are included as an important input to care via their role of monitoring health and progress, prevention, facilitating diagnosis and treatment and cooperating to assist the team in service delivery.

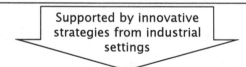

Supported by innovative strategies from industrial settings

Care Delivery Strategies Redefined

- Adopt a philosophy of zero defects;
- Restructure according to functional specialization; and
- Create goal-focused groups.

FIGURE 5.6   Medical Manufacturing in Clinical Settings

protocols as well as in the delivery of care rather than to exclude them. This will require a shift because in the past, physicians have made an effort to individualize patient treatment. When quality is measured by output, it becomes evident that the goal of including all patients within a set protocol produces the best results.

Thus, the goal of medical manufacturing is a consistent process that is understood and agreed upon by all the care providers forming the team. Patients need to understand the protocol and know why it was developed in a particular way and what the probabilities are for achieving the intended result if care is delivered accordingly. These ideas may tend to upset patients, physicians and medical group managers who believe that good results can never be achieved by a standardized process. That is why medical manufacturing is such a difficult undertaking. Those who resist this concept should examine the results from other settings. McDonald's has become famous for the high quality and consistency of its french fries, even when compared with french fries in some expensive restaurants. It is evident that many mass-produced manufactured goods (for example, french fries, cars, computers and so forth) can attain excellent quality despite standardization. This same phenomenon is possible in medical groups and in health care.

Medical Manufacturing Illustrated

A comparison between what presently happens in medical groups and what might happen under the concept of medical manufacturing illustrates the difference. A medical clinic's effort to diagnose and treat breast cancer provides a representative case study. Some assumptions must be made for this comparison. Approximately 12.5 percent of women will develop breast cancer. Assume there is a group of 100,000 patients being cared for by a large medical group and about 40,000 are women. Further assume that this patient cohort is stable over time and that susceptible women develop breast cancer over a 25-year period. If these assumptions hold true, there will be 5,000 breast cancer diagnoses for the cohort and about 200 cases will occur each year. If 100 primary physicians care for these women, then each physician will diagnose two breast cancers per year, or 50 breast cancers in 25 years.

Under a nonmedical manufacturing scenario, a patient has a mammogram once a year and sees the physician if she feels a lump in her breast. Her goal is to find breast cancer early and seek help so that it can be treated. The doctor's goal is the same. Assume that this woman examines her breasts regularly and eventually feels something about which she is concerned. She makes an appointment and sees her physician. The physician may have difficulty in detecting a mass and may tell her to come back in a month or, if concerned, may refer her to a surgeon for an examination. Sometimes the appointment is made concurrent with the time of diagnosis and sometimes the patient is instructed to make it after the visit of the diagnosis. The patient has a mammogram prior to visiting the surgeon. The surgeon may or may not be concerned. If concerned, further mammogram studies may be ordered and, if worrisome, a biopsy is done. Several weeks could easily transpire between the patient's first call to her physician and the biopsy.

If the biopsy is positive, the several-week delay is not the right thing done at the right time. Furthermore, the several-week interim period certainly is not kind. During this time the woman worries about cancer and dying; she is in limbo for several weeks about whether or not she will die. To be kind, this time period should not be longer than 36 hours, and preferably less. However, many in medicine today would say it is impossible to reduce the interim to 36 hours or less. Here is where medical manufacturing can be profitably applied.

If the concept of medical manufacturing were adopted, the 40,000 women would be treated quite differently. First, all 40,000 patients in our medical group's cohort would have yearly examinations. All breast problems and all aspects of diagnosis would be performed by one team for the clinic. Integral to this breast clinic would be the ability to have mammograms and biopsies; that is, all care would point to a definitive diagnosis. The team would be comprised of a few doctors, nurse practitioners, nurses, and educators. The team would be cohesive, have a rather flat organizational form, and be responsible for its own functioning. In other words, if a team member was not functioning effectively with others, his or her membership as a part of the team could be terminated. Under the medical manufacturing plan, the team will complete 40,000 breast examinations per year, diagnose 200 breast cancers, and gain valuable experience in reading mammograms and taking biopsies.

A patient who felt something in her breast could arrive at the clinic, have a mammogram, have it read immediately, have a breast examination and possibly even further tests the same day. The team would have decided on specific indications for biopsy. If an X-ray cone view of the breast were clinically necessary, it would be completed the same day or at least the next day. A biopsy and immediate frozen section could be completed within the same time parameters. Consequently, the patient would have an almost certain answer within *two days*. The process would be the same for all patients with the same signs and symptoms. If there were any delays in diagnosis, they would become evident quickly and the process could be modified. If some new knowledge developed that should change the process, the decision could be implemented easily.

SUPPORTIVE MEDICAL MANUFACTURING STRATEGIES

Zero Defects

An important goal for an enlightened medical group is to have no defects. With respect to breast cancer diagnosis, this would imply no delays in diagnosis and possibly from the patient's point of view, in a very strict sense, no deaths from breast cancer. However, in health care the ability to reach six sigma (that is, only 3.4 failures per million opportunities) is probably theoretical rather than practical because death for each of us is a certainty at some time. Nonetheless, we can do far better than we do now as far as quality control. Figure 5.6 suggests that a medical group using medical manufacturing might form an innovative strategy of zero defects.

Returning to our example, breast cancer is emerging as one of the greatest threats in health care from the viewpoint of legal liability. Patients are suing and winning when they get breast cancer. The team approach would provide increased safety in this respect. First, patients know the facts about the disease. They have contracted to do their own part in diagnosis (examination with monthly signed reports). Finally, all exams are identical and the diagnostic process is identical.

The team is performing 40,000 examinations per year with the diagnosis of 200 breast cancers. Each examiner is seeing about 30 patients per day and, if selected at random, would diagnose one cancer per week. All of this is performed under a strict protocol so that each examiner does the same thing with every patient. It should be very difficult to prove that there was any delay in diagnosis and that any misdiagnosis occurred. **The zero defect goal is important for patient care and is also important as protection against legal liability.**

Functional Specialization

A second innovative strategy consistent with medical manufacturing shown in Figure 5.6 is the idea of clustering patients who possess a common problem with the kinds of medical inputs necessary to provide the care. This is termed "functional specialization." In the early history of medical care, all physicians were generalists and did everything. As knowledge and skills increased, specialties evolved so that patients could receive better care. Some doctors took care of medical problems while others performed surgery. Thus, some of the specialties were separated by age of patient (pediatrics), anatomy (obstetrics and gynecology, gastroenterology), thinking (internal medicine) or doing (general surgery). Subspecialties developed as knowledge continued to increase.

With a growing intolerance for imperfect results and pressure to reduce cost, the demand grows for maximum expertise, standardization and lowest cost applied to every medical problem. There needs to be specialization by function where the necessary skills (and those providers who can apply them) are coordinated in a team approach for each large group of patients with the same problem. **Functional specialization then considers what group of providers (that is, teams) are necessary to deliver the care and implement the concept of medical manufacturing.** Also important is how the team will work together and the kind of power structure that will be the most effective in implementing the concept of medical manufacturing through functional specialization.

The example of diagnosing breast cancer can be further utilized in demonstrating the general concept of medical manufacturing. Figure 5.7 provides a comparative analysis of traditional functional approaches to care delivery for breast cancer. A common problem was chosen (that is, the diagnosis of breast problems), and from a functional perspective, a new specialist could be developed for this problem. In this case, several classical specialties are usually involved in the care of these patients. The initial exam is completed by a primary physician, the mammograms are read by a radiologist, and any abnormalities are sent to a surgeon for further diagnosis. Unless severe, a counselor is not involved for anxiety and there is seldom a proactive education program for patients to learn the facts about the diagnosis of breast cancer.

From a functional point of view, all of these aspects are necessary. Patients should know the facts and be informed that cooperation and active participation are necessary for good results. If an abnormality is discovered, all patients with that condition will be concerned about

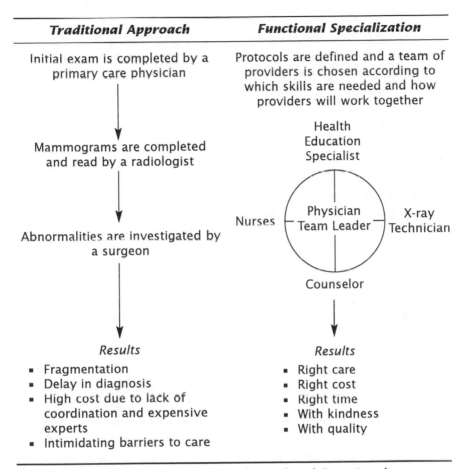

Traditional Approach	Functional Specialization
Initial exam is completed by a primary care physician	Protocols are defined and a team of providers is chosen according to which skills are needed and how providers will work together
Mammograms are completed and read by a radiologist	
Abnormalities are investigated by a surgeon	
Results	*Results*
• Fragmentation • Delay in diagnosis • High cost due to lack of coordination and expensive experts • Intimidating barriers to care	• Right care • Right cost • Right time • With kindness • With quality

FIGURE 5.7   A Comparison of Traditional and Functional Approaches to Care Delivery for Breast Cancer Detection

cancer and dying, so a counselor should be involved or at least available. Mammograms must be read accurately. An individual with maximum expertise must manage the examination and direction of the patient to the best protocol possible.

With functional specialization as shown in Figure 5.7, the goal is to have greater depth of knowledge in a narrower field while simultaneously lowering cost. In our illustration, maximum knowledge is desired about all aspects involved in the diagnosis of breast cancer as one narrow field. This is not beyond the capacity of one person. The team leader could be from any of the medical specialties. The depth of knowledge is important, not how this person was previously trained. In short, a specialist for the diagnosis of breast cancer would evolve. The benefits of this shift to functional specialization are apparent in comparison to the classical system of care where the diagnosis is haphazard, diagnosis and treatment are not standardized, care is fragmented and care is too expensive with only average results.

This proposal for specialization might horrify some physicians. Their immediate response will be that only a board-qualified radiologist can read mammograms, that only a board-certified surgeon can do a breast biopsy and that general surgeons should not waste their time examining patients. It is interesting to note that in many cases today, an ultrasound machine completes the biopsy when someone flips a switch. Yes, in many institutions, surgeons and radiologists are arguing over who should flip the switch and who should get the surgical fee. With respect to mammograms, all radiologists have had to learn to read them within the last decade.

Functional specialization should be considered whenever a certain clinical problem is frequent and requires the consultation of two or more specialists. In these situations, for greater productivity, the clinical problems should be analyzed to determine whether one of the specialists or a single doctor (or other professional) could provide the maximum expertise for the entire clinical problem. This would increase productivity and avoid a reduction in fees. Increasing productivity is a promising way to reduce costs, retain quality and avoid a broad-scale reduction in all fees paid to health care personnel. Medical groups in the health care field must consider the same technologies that have motivated business for years. **That is why the term "medical manufacturing" is being proposed to help physicians and medical groups understand that they should adopt practices that have proven successful in intensely competitive settings.**

Goal-Focused Groups

Goal-focused groups is a third strategy for innovating under medical manufacturing. Applying the medical manufacturing concept for common clinical entities, rather strict protocols can be developed with the right thing at the right time at effective cost and kindness as the goal. Functional specialization provides an infrastructure for medical manufacturing, and goal-focused groups or teams provide a means for implementation.

The wide range of organizational designs and authority relationships in health care are legendary. There are hierarchical HMO structures, hospital structures and professional structures. In medicine, there are specialty departments and family practice departments. There is nursing with a vertical department structure and, if present, education and counseling also have their own structures. Health care protocols are being developed by doctors in specialty departments, but they are often the sum of what each doctor wants rather than a simplified, single pathway. This creates further structures. Nursing develops protocols for the problem that may or may not fit with the doctors' protocol. Hospital administration adds some requirements, and the final product often has no possibility of effective function (Tjosvold & MacPherson, 1996). Worst of all, protocols are meant to give some medical-legal protection but, in fact, accomplish the opposite because no one can or does follow the protocols. The excessive proliferation of structure explains why a cohesive, multispecialty team is necessary to implement the concept of medical manufacturing (Pauly, 1996).

For clinical problems, a multispecialty approach could be adopted as appropriate involving case managers, doctors, nurses, and clinical specialists. Depending on the clinical problem, the team might add nurse practitioners, medical assistants, counselors, or educators. The goal-focused group determines what functions are necessary and then adjusts the structure secondary to the function. This approach conflicts with the past heritage in medicine wherein a structure was adopted and then adjusted to fit the function. Now, function will come first and the structure will support the function.

The traditional tendency to rely on structure explains why a cohesive, multispecialty team is necessary to implement the concept of medical manufacturing. The building blocks of goal-focused groups are illustrated in Figure 5.8. A group compromised of providers with skills pertinent to all facets of a common clinical problem should be established. There should be a representative for all aspects of the clinical problem. However, to the extent that different components of the clinical problem can be combined in one individual, productivity will be increased and costs reduced. The team needs to consider the classical problem and produce one protocol (although there may be clearly defined variations) that can and will be followed by the entire team. Care in the office, diagnostic areas or in the hospital must be coordinated under the direction of the team.

Block #1

Characteristics of Goal-Focused Groups

Cohesive, multispecialty group comprised of care delivery personnel who possess skills and experience pertinent to all facets of a clinical problem

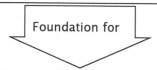

Foundation for

Block #2

Group Process

- Input on clinical problem is enhanced by representation from the diverse team.
- Protocol is defined by all the team members.
- Care delivery is coordinated by the team.
- Evaluation and control are reinforced in order to fine-tune the protocol and to improve team functioning.

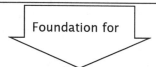

Foundation for

Block #3

Issues Refinement in Implementation

- No team member is asked to do something that he or she does not know how to do or for which expertise cannot be developed.
- Team members share ideas to improve team functioning.
- Relative contribution and cost ratios are analyzed to achieve the best cost care by the most appropriate provider.

Figure 5.8   The Building Blocks of Goal-Focused Groups

After the team has developed a protocol, it must adopt the six-sigma approach and simplify the protocol again, keeping in mind that the ultimate objective is the highest-quality care. This is possible if quality is measured by output and is impossible if quality is measured by process. The team must again review the specific problem. Does this protocol specifically address the problem and is the goal clear? A definitive endpoint is necessary if the team is to reach it. Then, considerable attention needs to be given to what kind of a team is necessary.

Peter Drucker, in *Post Capitalist Society(1993),* describes three kinds of teams. For high productivity, a team must be organized that is appropriate to the work. The first type of team is exemplified by a baseball team. Each player has a fixed position and a fixed function, and the performance of each can be measured. Part of a surgical team in a hospital performs the same way as a baseball team. Individual players form this first kind of team, but they do not necessarily function as a team. The second type of team is exemplified by a soccer team, an orchestra or an emergency department team in a cardiac arrest. Again, players have fixed positions; but here the members are both on the team and function as a team. There is, however, much more flexibility of position than is true in the baseball team. The third type of team is exemplified by doubles in tennis. Although the players have preferred positions, they are not fixed. They cover for each other and adjust for the strengths and weaknesses of each other. This team only really functions best over a period of time when learning how to adjust for the respective strengths and weaknesses of each team member as a conditioned reflex. Change from one kind of team to another is difficult, and the change disrupts long established-relationships and time-honored ways of function.

In medicine, there is a fourth type of team: an ad hoc grouping that is temporary so that the group is a team in name only. Members are not on a stable team and, thus, cannot begin to function as a team. For example, the anesthesiologist would not become a member of the surgical team. However, the surgeon and his or her assistants would ideally function more like the tennis doubles. To some extent this would include the scrub nurse.

However, there is a major problem with the ad hoc team that can be called the "interface problem." Doctors are in one group, nurses are in another and surgical assistants (that is, residents, scrub technicians) are often in another. All of these groups rotate, so that at any given time, the team (but not really a team) taking care of the patient is an ad hoc group coming together at that moment. None of the individuals is strictly on a team and, thus, the group has no possibility of functioning as a team. It is similar to the situation in which all the baseball players in the American or National leagues are shuffled and assigned to a new team each day. Each individual would have a fixed position, but the group would not be able to play as well as an intact baseball team. They would not be a team even though they were labeled as such.

The experience of most businesses in changing from the first type of team (that is, strict functional specialization) to the second type of team (team-based specialization) has been advantageous. It can be strongly argued that this model would be very applicable in health care under medical manufacturing. For a given clinical problem as suggested in Figure 5.8, the team members would leave behind their past allegiance to administration, nursing or medicine. They would substitute allegiance to the clinical process and to the team. As discussed in Sidebar 5.5, implementing goal-focused groups is not always problem-free.

In the example of the team developed for breast cancer diagnosis, there is both an educational function and a counseling function that must be recognized due to patients' false expectations of perfection and the stress of possible cancer. The goal-focused group can incorporate these functions, as shown in Figure 5.8. These functions could be performed by educators and counselors, or it might be more effective to have nurses provide this care.

For a clinical team, a physician will probably be the team leader. This leader needs to be aware of and sympathetic to all the various functions of the team; that is, both a respected clinician and leader. The goal-focused team will challenge many of the traditions in medicine. Mid-level providers such as nurse practitioners (and certified nurse midwives) should be given authority to see patients alone without direct supervision. In other words, they perform tasks more independently than nurses traditionally perform. They may replace physicians on a team in order to pursue cost effectiveness. To be cost effective, nurse practitioners should not simply be hired to assist physicians.

Nurses can function independently as care providers to a far greater extent than most physicians realize. If a team is to function effectively, nurses should be given this latitude. Nurses have assumed increased responsibility in doctors' offices for years but have been strictly regi-

SIDEBAR 5.5

Issues in Implementing Goal-Focused Teams

When considering what each member of the team should do, several general issues surface during implementation. First, no team member should be asked to perform a task that he or she does not know how to do. Moreover, everyone should stay within their skill, capability, experience and knowledge. This requires integrity and self-awareness. Adequate and ongoing training should be available for every clinical function. Second, ideally, members of the team will constantly bring back ideas and suggestions for better team function. If some procedure is considered for adoption, all team members must be equally prepared. This may imply using a consultant for training or assigning a team member to learn the skills prior to teaching the other members. In this manner, all team members can reach a functional capacity that is their maximum rather than a minimum.

An example of appropriate task assignment for a nurse practitioner is evident in gynecology. In a busy office for routine gynecological examinations, an experienced doctor might complete an exam every 15 minutes, or four in an hour. Some patients will need to talk longer. Nurse practitioners can do these exams independently and consult only if necessary. Suppose a nurse took a history, did the pelvic examination, prescribed the medication, if any, and the doctor entered the care delivery process at the end in an oversight function. The doctor could be given a report, sign the prescription and probably manage two or three nurses in the course of this process. Thus, the doctor might effectively see 10 to 12 patients per hour. Many physicians would object that a nurse could not do a satisfactory pelvic examination, but in labor and delivery, nurses routinely perform pelvic examinations on patients in labor (which is more difficult) and make diagnoses (which are more critical).

A third issue to consider in the implementation of goal-focused groups concerns staff management. To achieve maximum productivity and lowest cost, the delivery of care should be performed by the lowest-cost, but qualified, staff member. A rough estimate of cost (salaries) of various personnel might be as follows:

Provider	Weighted Cost	Provider	Weighted Cost
Nurse	X	Educator	X
Nursepractitioner	2X	Counselor	1.5X
Physician	8X	Clerical	.7X

continued

To achieve the highest productivity and lowest cost of care implies caring for the maximum number of patients at the minimum cost while at the same time fulfilling the goal of performing the right care at the right time with kindness—and not rationing care. To do this, personnel must be used effectively. Nurses should not do clerical work, nurse practitioners should not do nurses' work, and doctors should not perform the tasks that nurse practitioners or nurses can do. If there is cost effectiveness, the cost of care should be reduced with the savings passed on to the patient and team members.

There are problems with this medical manufacturing proposal just as there are problems with any new way of doing things. Each team will have several doctors, and they all need to function together clinically and emotionally. The lack of hierarchy may create a problem. In resolving these problems, each team member should feel free to make a suggestion that will be respected and given equal weight. Doctors in the past have delivered the entire care for each patient. **In the future, their role should be to enable the care to be provided rather than to provide all the care themselves.**

---

mented in hospitals. In hospitals they observe, complete assessments and carry out orders. However, in two clinical areas, close observation shows that nurses have made diagnoses, instituted treatment and taken far more responsibility than is generally acknowledged.

One area is the surgical recovery room. Here, nurses receive immediate postoperative patients, constantly assess their condition and respond to the patients' needs. Doctors are available, but many decisions are made without consultation. For example, at night, one patient may be postoperative in the recovery room with the anesthesiologist and surgeon. The recovery room nurse is essentially alone. Another area of increased responsibility is labor and delivery. Here again, nurses are often alone with patients at night without a doctor in the hospital. They must assess the patient, provide pain medication as indicated, consult when necessary and call the obstetrician when appropriate. At times, they must diagnose and treat an emergency until the doctor arrives.

APPLICATIONS FOR MANAGERS

The essence of a true increase in productivity in medical practice will rest on zero defects, functional specialization, and collaborative practice—programmatic-level strategies supporting an effort at medical manufacturing. These are the primary methods of dramatically increasing productivity without reducing quality. However, these strategies depend upon a minimal patient volume and clustering similar patients. This is a shift in approach to care delivery. This approach could never be considered in the past because patients were not clustered. Patients came one-by-one to each doctor. Now, with managed care in the ascendancy, similar patients can be clustered together by medical groups.

Physicians have delivered the entire care for each patient in the past. In the future, their role will shift to enabling care rather than providing all the care themselves. If these proposals (and others) under medical manufacturing—zero defects, functional specialization and goal-focused teams—could be implemented, the cost of caring for a specific patient cohort could be reduced substantially without reducing the remuneration of any personnel. The gain would be possible by increasing productivity, reducing personnel and coordinating the entire process in the most effective manner.

Throughout recent efforts at improving the health care delivery system, there continues to surface a discouraging realization. Despite our best efforts to address rising health costs and the creation of innovative policies, the results fall short of the expectations. The answer to why these shortcomings occur can be attributed to a piecemeal approach that resolves one issue at a time without regard for the whole problem. We have enough experience with these incremental resolutions to realize that they will not accomplish what needs to be achieved—systematic reform. Addressing one piece of the puzzle only to overlook other pieces, or to exacerbate the entire puzzle, will not lead to the answers that are vitally needed in the health care system.

There are too many examples from the field of business to believe that a naïve, incremental approach will solve the problems. Businesses that are besieged by foreign competition recognize that survival means pulling out all the stops; halfway remedies will not work. Corporations have responded to intensifying competition through innovation and widespread reengineering. Health care, in the meanwhile, continues to tinker at the margins. Excessive regulations, professional control and similar constraints are preventing this nation from instilling the degree of change so vitally needed to save one of the world's best sources of medical expertise. At this point, a revolution may be necessary to avoid sinking any further into a lethal implosion.

Against this backdrop is the promising opportunity for medical groups to rise above the traditional constraints and incremental approaches by adopting proven methods for organizing and delivering care. Many of the most fruitful strategies are found in business. The transition to medical manufacturing may not sound very appealing to medical groups or to physicians who will discover a radically new practice context upon adopting the strategies. However, medical groups still have the luxury of voluntarily embracing these techniques to their advantage. Unless powerful alterations are adopted, the final outcome may result in significant constraints on medical practice and the very delivery of care.

REFERENCES

Arndt, M., & Bigelow, B. (1998). Reengineering: Déjà vu all over again. *Health Care Management Review, 23*(3), 58–66.

Bachman, M. A. (1997, January/February). The physician office laboratory: Profitability under managed care. *MGM Journal,* 28–31.

Cleverley, W. O. (1995). Understanding your hospital's true financial position and changing it. *Health Care Management Review, 20*(2), 62–73.

Conrad, D. A., Maynard C., Cheadle A., Ramsey S., Marcus-Smith M., Kirz, Madden, C. A., Martin D., Perrin, E. B., Wickizer T., Zierler B., Ross A., Norb, Liang S. Y. (1998, March 18). Primary care physician compensation method in medical groups. *Journal of the American Medical Association, 279*(11), 853–858.

De Angelo, L. (1995, November/December). Collaborative practice. *MGM Journal,* 12–16, 85.

Dixon, R., & Trenchard, P. M. (1996). The role of precision and quality in clinical costings. *Health Care Management Review, 21*(2), 7–15.

Drucker, P. F. (1993). *Post-capitalist society.* New York: Harper Business.

Gamm, L. D. (1996). Dimensions of accountability for not-for-profit hospitals and health systems. *Health Care Management Review, 21*(2), 87–95.

Gold, M. (1997). Markets and public programs: Insight from Oregon and Tennessee. *Journal of Health Politics, Policy and Law, 22*(2), 633–666.

Greene, B. R. (1996). Understanding the forces driving medical group practice activities: An overview. *Journal of Ambulatory Care Management, 19*(4), 1–3.

Ho, S. K., Chan, L., & Kidwell, R. E. (1999). The implementation of business process reengineering in American and Canadian hospitals. *Health Care Management Review, 24*(2), 19–31.

Iglehart, J. K. (1995, Summer). A new era: Modest reform and managed care. *Health Affairs,* 5–6.

Johnson, E. A. (1995). The public's future perspective on managed care. *Health Care Management Review, 20*(2), 45–47.

Kertesz, L. (1998, March 16). Cost-control burden on HMOs' shoulders. *Modern Healthcare,* 78–80.

Krentz, S. E. (1997, May). Maximizing financial returns by meeting employer expectations. *Healthcare Financial Management,* 45–47.

Lowes, R. L. (1998, April 13). Making midlevel providers click with your group. *Medical Economics,* 123–132.

Olden, P. C. (1996, May/June). Managing the managed care market competition. *MGM Journal,* 15–22.

Pauly, M. V. (1996). Economics of multispecialty group practice. *Journal of Ambulatory Care Management, 19*(3), 26–33.

Preston, S. H. (1997, July 14). Adding profitable services that fit your practice. *Medical Economics,* 81–96.

Ryan, J. B., & Clay, S. B. (1995, October). Understanding the law of large numbers. *Healthcare Financial Management, 49*(10): 22, 24.

Smith, H. L., Yourstone, S. A., Lorber, D., & Mann, B. (2001). Managed care and medical practice guidelines: The thorny problem of attaining physician compliance. *Advances in Health Care Management, 2,* 93–130.

Tjosvold, D., & MacPherson, R. C. (1996). Joint hospital management by physicians and nursing administrators. *Health Care Management Review, 21*(3), 43–54.

Trauner, J. B., & Chesnutt, J. S. (1996). Medical groups in California: Managing care under capitation. *Health Affairs, 15*(1), 159–170.

Van Horn, R. L., Burns, L. R., & Wholey, D. R. (1997). The impact of physician involvement in managed care on efficient use of hospital resources. *Medical Care, 35*(9), 873–889.

Washburn, E. R. (1995, July/August). Budgeting for a more likely future. *MGM Journal,* 74–78.

Wood, K .M., & Matthews, G. E. (1997, July). Reviewing practice expenses can improve profitability. *Healthcare Financial Management, 51*(7): 81–83.

Yasin, M. M., Czuchry, A. J., Jennings, D. L. & York, C. (1999). Managing the quality effort in a health care setting. *Health Care Management Review, 24*(1), 45–56.

Zwanziger, J., & Melnick, G. A. (1996). Can managed care plans control health care costs. *Health Affairs, 15*(2), 185–199.

Chapter 6

The Assurance of High-Quality Care

Executive Summary

Delivering the right care at the right time with kindness and caring is only relevant if that care is also of high quality. But what is "high-quality care"? Although consumers (and many providers) are unable to precisely define what they mean by quality care, this does not prevent them from forming important perceptions about care with less-than-perfect information. Medical groups can respond significantly to this vacuum of knowledge through leadership in developing a quality management program.

Low-quality care and service delivery only generate adaptive responses by consumers (and their lawyers), and governmental and not-for-profit accrediting organizations through litigation, regulation and legislation. Seldom do these responses lead to more efficient care delivery in attaining the objective of enhanced quality. More often than not, these responses create perturbations that further constrain conscientious efforts at controlling quality.

Medical groups must address five rationales that lead patients to initiate litigation for poor outcomes:

- Incorrect expectations;
- Unanticipated complications;
- Unexpected results or misunderstanding about proposed care;
- Lack of patient partnerships in decision making; and
- Lack of perceived consent.

This chapter proposes that rigorous and innovative quality assurance programs can help to minimize these problems. However, it is necessary to draw deeply upon principles of continuous quality improvement long utilized in business.

Several suggestions for medical groups to consider in developing continuous improvement programs are considered, including:

- Informing medical, nursing and administrative staff about differences in perspective on dimensions of quality;
- Reaching a definition of quality of care based upon efforts by the Joint Commission on Accreditation of Healthcare Organizations and existing health care research;
- Adopting reengineering practices; and
- Using clinical and outcomes benchmarks and best practices.

These strategies form a base from which medical groups can significantly affect service delivery.

THE UNINFORMED CONSUMER

Of the many purchases that consumers make, health care expenditures are made with surprising ignorance. There is simply a shortage of worthwhile, comparable information on managed care plans and on specific physicians (Spragins, 1999). Consequently, even if the public wished to shop wisely among health plans, health facilities and clinicians, there are no benchmark data easily available for comparative purposes. For most material expenditures—land, housing, automobiles, appliances, electronic products, entertainment goods—a consumer can readily turn to a wide variety of reliable sources for information. Yet, for the very important decisions about which managed care plan and which physician(s) to partner with in remaining healthy, the consumer has virtually no information. It is easier to ascertain the value of a six-pack of soda pop than it is to understand the comparative advantages and disadvantages of two managed care plans.

Due to the need to establish basic information to facilitate consumer choice and to set standards for care delivery, the National Commission on Quality Assurance (NCQA) has attempted to gather performance measures from HMOs. The not-for-profit NCQA has created a Quality Compass to assess plan performance across many clinical areas. Unfortunately, of the 447 health plans that provide information to the Quality Compass database, only 292, or 65 percent, have agreed to disclose their performance. Thus, consumers can only speculate about some comparisons among plans. The reluctance of 35 percent of responding HMOs to disclose their performance under Quality Compass raises serious questions about what the plans may be hiding. At the very least, consumers have a difficult time knowing which managed care plans are providing high quality of care.

A reinvented health care system must provide the assurance of high-quality care for consumers. Health care that can only boast about low costs will miss an essential part of the consumer's value equation (Eddy, 1997). Each consumer has a unique formula, or perspective, on the proper mix of cost and quality. Consumers may not be able to articulate their preferred balance, but they do know it when they see it. Researchers in this area argue that the majority of consumers are seeking an unusual balance in that they want an unrealistically high level of quality for minimal cost. Thus, providers face a significant dilemma for the future in convincing consumers (and usually the employers that select managed care plans for consumer choice) that they can deliver quality services within reasonable pricing parameters (Kuttner, 1998).

Figure 6.1 illustrates several potential reactions by patients and consumers when they do not, or perceive that they do not, receive high-quality health care. The challenge for health care providers is to deliver seamless services of such high quality that consumers have no reason to react adversely. Some would say that this ability to achieve zero defects in health care is unrealistic because medicine blends both art and science. However, leading corporations throughout the world have rigorously pursued the concept of zero defects even though they are producing millions of products or serving millions of customers.

Before considering the strategies that managed care plans might follow in achieving business-like standards for quality, it is appropriate to first examine the reactions of consumers to what they perceive to be low-quality health care. As Figure 6.1 suggests, there are at least two types of errors that cause dissatisfaction among patients. First,

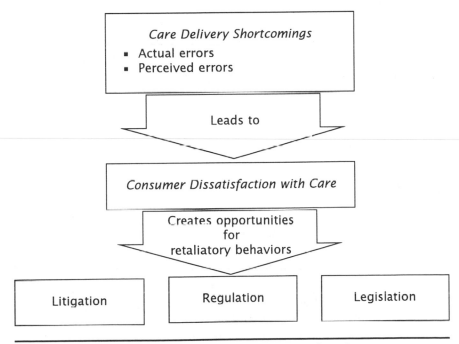

FIGURE 6.1 Consumer Reactions to Poor-Quality Care

there are actual errors that lead to higher morbidity and mortality. The precise rate of errors is not known, but estimates offer chilling testimony, as suggested in Sidebar 6.1.

The second type of error leading to patient dissatisfaction pertains to perceptions. In these instances, the health care provider may have followed all of the correct protocols surrounding the episode. However, the patient erroneously perceives that a mistake has been made. Even though the provider is not at fault, the patient persists in perceiving that an error was made. The end result can be the same as that for an actual error.

ADAPTIVE RESPONSES TO LOW QUALITY OF CARE

Figure 6.1 implies that consumers can implement a number of adaptive responses to their perceptions of low-quality care delivered by health care organizations. In effect, the failure to deliver care that satisfies the end user creates opportunities for retaliatory behavior by consumers and consumer groups. Litigation, or malpractice litigation, is the individual consumer's greatest weapon against poor-quality health care. There is an entire industry of professionals waiting to assist consumers in their efforts to derive justice from the legal system. Medical malpractice has driven up the cost of care as physicians and other providers cover their bases with substantial testing in order to avoid high risk/exposure (Huntington, 1998). Regulation and legislation are the two weapons against poor-quality health care that are invoked on behalf of large groups of consumers. Health care has been governed by high levels of legislation and ensuing regulations flowing from enacted legislation.

LITIGATION

Historically, medical practice has been based on diagnosing and treating patients' problems. From symptoms and physical examination, a diagnosis was made and the patient was provided with the best treatment for the diagnosis. Until the last century, the best treatment was often just being kind to the patient and relieving suffering. Recently, there has been an explosion of scientific knowledge and a plethora of effective treatments. This has been good for the patient, but as better treatments were discovered, some of the caring has dis-

Sidebar 6.1

System Errors as a Prevalent Health Care Delivery Phenomenon

Errors in health care systems are not widely reported; however, a number of research studies shed some light on the magnitude of system errors occurring in health care delivery. Leape (1994) reviewed several studies of error rates in medicine. It is estimated that 36 percent of all patients admitted to a teaching hospital experienced an iatrogenic event (Steel, Gertman, Crescenzi, & Anderson, 1981). Leape also reviewed the 1991 Harvard Medical Practice Study that reported the results of a population-based study of iatrogenic injury in patients hospitalized in New York State in 1984. The findings are alarming because nearly 4 percent of all patients suffered an injury that prolonged their stay or resulted in measurable disability. For New York State, this equaled 98,609 patients in 1984, and nearly 14 percent of these injuries resulted in a fatality. Leape observes that if these rates are typical of those of the United States, then 180,000 people die each year partly as a result of iatrogenic injury. This is the equivalent of three jumbo-jet crashes every two days; an error rate that is intolerable in transportation but apparently acceptable in health care.

The Harvard Medical Practice Study discovered that about 1 million potentially preventable medical errors result in 120,000 deaths each year (Leape, Lawthers, Brennan, & Johnson, 1993). Despite the magnitude of the problem, the routine occurrence of systematic error is probably not clear to many health care administrators. According to Leape and colleagues, ". . . most doctors and hospitals really don't know how many errors they have. The reason is quite simple. We rely almost entirely on self-report" (Leape et al., 1993). The costs associated with these preventable errors has not been estimated, but they must be enormous. However, health care managers may discover that medical practice errors and their costs only represent the tip of the iceberg in terms of systematic errors accompanying health care delivery.

Lesar, Briceland and Stein (1997) reported on the primary factors accompanying errors in medication prescriptions. Knowledge-based errors in drug therapy accounted for 30 percent of all errors in a 631-bed tertiary care teaching hospital over a one-year period. Knowledge-based errors concerning patient factors that affect drug therapy accounted for 29.2 percent of the errors in this hospital. Use of calculations, decimal points, rate or unit expression factors accounted for 17.5 percent of errors. Incorrect

continued

drug names, abbreviations and dosages accounted for 13.4 percent of errors. Insights on the cost of these errors associated with medication surfaced in another hospital study. Bates and associates (1997) estimated that the annual costs attributable for all adverse drug events and preventable adverse drug events at a 700-bed teaching hospital were $5.6 million and $2.8 million, respectively. **In sum, many health care delivery errors spanning a wide array of patient care services may present a cost that is simply intolerable in this era of fiscal constraints.**

appeared. This has affected the ideal, close relationship between the doctor and the patient and, in turn, has contributed to the rise in malpractice litigation.

The opportunity for malpractice litigation arose because some physicians attempted to deliver care that, frankly, should not have been attempted due to shortcomings in skill levels and ability. In other instances, there was a deliberate attempt to pursue a goal other than providing the best treatment, such as performing operations in order to make money rather than helping the patient. Although rare, these undeserved medical care events have happened over the history of medicine. Malpractice has been effective in instilling control over these abuses. However, the malpractice concept has subsequently been extended to include any bad results in care delivery regardless of whether or not there was intent to harm.

Medical practice, like investing or sports, is not an exact science. Patients are not always better after receiving treatment, and sometimes they are physically or mentally worse for the care they have received. One can never be certain that the tried-and-true treatment for a given malady will result in the improvement of every patient. There may be unanticipated results. Moreover, there may be several equally accepted treatments from which physicians must choose. Innate skill and judgment have been the basis for sorting among these alternative medical decisions. Increasingly, laboratory tests are assuming a more important role in diagnosis and treatment. However, the art of medical practice remains a dominant aspect that contributes to malpractice risk. Malpractice appears to be pursued by patients in response to unanticipated results that upset them even when appropriate skill and judgment were used.

The tendency for patients to sue over unanticipated results appears to be unique to medicine. In other professional endeavors, there is a limited proclivity to use litigation solely due to unanticipated results. For example, at one time most furniture was made entirely by hand, reflecting craftsmanship and skill of the industrial artisan. Chippendale, for example, proved over the years to be a genius while others were not nearly as good in producing high-quality furniture. However, the lesser craftsmen were not threatened with lawsuits simply because they were not as good as Chippendale. Alternatively, consider the area of investing. Brokers are typically not sued because their recommended mutual funds do not perform as well as other investments. This assumes, of course, that no attempt has been made to swindle. In retrospect, one can always argue that a fund manager should have done something else to earn money on an investment, but the investment manager is generally protected from litigation because of the hundreds of extraneous factors influencing a given investment. The same phenomenon occurs in athletic contests. There are winners and losers, but coaches and team members are not sued simply because they lost. In retrospect, it is often obvious that the game could have been played in a different, more effective way. Nonetheless, the coaches and players are not held liable for poor results.

The pursuit of legal action by patients due to a bad result is, in some respects, less disruptive for clinicians than the recognition that litigation may occur. Legal action is feared by the medical and health care establishment. This fear is associated with a little understood facet of behavior; that is, to effectively modify or change behavior, two prerequisites are necessary: The reward or punishment must be significant and the significant reward or punishment must be capricious. One of the best examples is gambling. Many individuals gamble when they cannot afford to lose any money. There is always the possibility of a large win (that is, a significant reward) and the results of gambling are capricious. Although the chances of a large win are small, it is distributed according to chance and therefore cannot be predicted.

The opposite of the reward principle is also true. For example, it is generally believed that punishment will deter crime. Although the punishment may be severe, it may not be capricious and therefore does not modify behavior. In other countries, behavior is modified because the punishment is both severe and capricious. This is the reason that legal liability in this country is beginning to have a marked effect on the practice of medicine. The legal suit is considered severe by the plaintiff (the doctor) and the results are capricious. The fact that the doctor may have adequate insurance and good legal representation is immaterial; there is the fear of a trial and the possibility that insurance will be subsequently canceled.

Legal liability and malpractice are also closely related to informed consent. Some history is important to understand the changing perspectives about informed consent. At one time when there was an established doctor-patient relationship, patients considered doctors experts and just did as they advised. As treatments and operations became more complex, patients deserved to know more about the possible dangers and results (Hickson, Clayton, Githerns, & Sloan, 1992). As a result, patients began to sue for malpractice on the basis that they had not known or been told about possible results of the treatment. At times, they sued even when the treatment had been successful in delivering a cure (for example, surgical removal of cancer) but had left them somewhat disabled or disfigured.

Even the best doctors have difficulty with informed consent as it is emerging (Adamson, Tschann, Guillion, & Oppenberg, 1989). In some situations, they assume the patient knows that treatment is dangerous or damaging (for example, radiation for cancer) to some extent. At other times it is difficult to know whether the remotest dangers should be discussed (that is, there is the possibility of death with any operation). Furthermore, what is to be done when a patient refuses the best and least dangerous treatment because of an unrealistic fear? Can the patient dictate a more serious treatment that is objectively more dangerous? From a legal point of view, all of these trends may be converging. If so, they will have an enormous impact on medicine and health care.

The fundamental effect has been an increase in excessive caution among physicians. For example, there has been much publicity about mothers and new babies leaving the hospital in 24 hours or less after delivery. In selected cases, this is probably safe for the mother because she will know how she feels and can access care if anything changes. The early discharge is partially motivated by saving money, but one cannot totally predict the future of newborns at 24 hours. Some will get into trouble at 36 or 48 hours, and a new mother might not pick up early signs of trouble. Think of the results if a newborn had problems at 36 hours that were not recognized. The providers would be successfully sued for early discharge. As an extension of the concept of informed consent, the mother should have been told that insurance would not pay for another day in the hospital and that there was the possibility of trouble with the baby at 36 hours. If the mother did not return immediately in these situations, the baby could die.

The trends in legal liability with respect to untoward outcomes and informed consent will have a huge impact on how medicine is practiced. As a result, those involved in decision making have a powerful impetus to modify the practice of medicine and the delivery of health care to protect themselves. Malpractice tends to reduce the value of judgment. If the results are not perfect, it would tend to show that a provider's judgment was poor. Therefore, medicine searches for more concrete evidence of good intent. Here, the concept of implied certainty is important. If someone performs a laboratory test with the results expressed in a number, the quantitative value (whether positive or negative) appears to have greater certainty. In contrast, when a provider issues a professional opinion based on good judgment and years of experience, it may, in fact, be the absolute truth. The number from a test may be based on a faulty procedure and can be wrong. Nevertheless, the number appears to have greater certainty. Thus, tests are increasingly used in medicine because, from a legal point of view, there seems to be more proof.

As health care changes to protect the provider and prove good intent, more tests will be used and the judgment of experts will be reduced in value. When considering possible ways to protect against legal action, a complication that occurs one in 1,000 times may be given the same weight as one that occurs once in 20 times. The strength of a chain is actually based on the weakest link. In a medical chain, often there are links that cannot be made stronger. The solution seems to be to make the stronger links stronger even though there is one link that cannot be changed. This is unproductive and expensive but seems to give the impression that everything was done that could have been done.

From this discussion, it is evident that many of the factors encouraging malpractice litigation are not primarily concerned with better care for the patient and certainly not with the most effective care considering cost. Solutions will be difficult. Litigation over the years in medicine has helped to correct some injustice and bad practice. However, frivolous litigation tends to devalue judgment and make health care much more expensive due to defensive medicine.

Attacking the Heart of Malpractice Litigation

The structure, process and outcomes of care delivery and patient-systems design efforts are crucial with respect to managing malpractice. One of the things that generates anger among patients is the feeling that they have been treated unjustly or unfairly (Sloan, Mergenhagen, Burfield, Bovbjerg, & Hassen, 1989). The restructuring of managed care and medical practice over the last 10 years has made patients more susceptible to feeling that the system has been unjust, unfair or simply incompetent. Often, angry patients do not have anyone in the system they can talk to, especially if their primary care physician has made them angry. From the patient's view, the system may tell them everything has been perfect when their perceived reality is quite the converse.

Consider the case of the patient who recently changed her HMO because her employer switched to a new managed care provider. Previously, she had seen a specific internist and a gynecologist. She was told about primary care physicians with whom she could form a relationship and that they would be available and help her navigate the system to receive the finest care. She was given a list of 20 primary care physicians and told she could choose one that she liked. It was suggested she interview several and choose one. It turned out that 18 of the primary care physicians had closed panels, so she effectively had a choice of two. Furthermore, unless she had an emergency, both of the two primary care physicians available could not see her for a month.

From the patient's point of view, she had to give up seeing specialists that she knew and liked. From a retrospective point of view, the provider availability options from the HMO were false; the actual situation was not at all like the one described. Effectively, the patient had little choice and no advocate. It was natural that she would feel unfairly treated. One could not plan a better precursor for a subsequent malpractice suit if the patient is not satisfied with medical care in the future.

Legal action for adverse clinical outcomes is pursued for a number of reasons, such as:

- Incorrect expectations;
- Unanticipated complications;

- Unexpected results or misunderstanding regarding proposed care;
- Lack of patient partnerships in decision making; and
- Lack of perceived consent.

Efforts by medical groups and providers to address the malpractice situation should concentrate on these five general reasons why patients may initiate legal action.

Incorrect Expectations

Incorrect expectations form one of the most important causal factors for malpractice litigation (Entman et al., 1994). The significance of realistic expectations is evident in all aspects of our lives. Fast-food chains do not make the best hamburgers in the world, but people are usually satisfied because they know what to expect, a consistent product is delivered, and the food is not expensive. If a consumer went to an expensive restaurant and received the same hamburger, fury would result because the expectation would be a much better hamburger cooked to exact specifications (that is, rare, medium or well done).

Unanticipated Complications

Individuals may become angry about complications. Most treatments in medical practice have some complications. Patients may be unaware because they were not told or because they did not want to hear what their provider was telling them. After an operation, they may have an infection or have more pain than expected. The solution for better understanding is to create a system wherein providers can evaluate what the patient knows or expects and then educate in a gentle way. One person, the doctor, cannot do this effectively from either a time or a perspective point of view. The crucial factor is that the patient really understands and acknowledges the truth concerning all facets of the treatment. No provider is able to conclude unequivocally that a specific intervention is in a patient's best interest.

Unexpected Results or Misunderstanding about Proposed Care

There may be unexpected results and misunderstanding about all facets of the proposed care. For example, a woman in her forties needs a hysterectomy. The question arises as to whether or not her ovaries should be removed. Removal means that normal tissue will be taken and that the woman will need to take estrogen. If the ovaries are removed, the woman will not get ovarian cancer in the future. This is a fairly common, highly lethal form of cancer. Moreover, for most women, the ovaries will cease to function in a few years and then estrogen will be necessary anyway. Doctors practice both ways. Some physicians feel ovaries should be removed when childbearing is finished. Others believe normal tissue should not necessarily be removed. The crucial aspect with respect to malpractice is that the patient should understand the pros and cons of each path, be a full partner in the decision and discuss the decision in a relaxed atmosphere. Decisions of this type are best made in discussion with several informed individuals; not with one doctor who maintains a strict, doctrinaire position. Above all, it is essential to avoid the situation wherein the patient claims after the operation that she did not realize that she would need to take estrogen after the surgery.

Lack of Patient Partnerships in Decision Making

The concept of the patient being a full partner in decisions about care is very important. To do this, the patient must be knowledgeable about his or her condition before a decision is made. Becoming knowledgeable about a personal health problem requires education and discussion over time. Then, when a decision is to be made, the patient can be a true partner. In the classical approach to medical practice, a proposed course of treatment is suggested, and then the patient is told about alternatives. In many cases, this situation presents too much information in too short a time for the patient to really take an active part in the decision-making process. Physicians and medical groups can alternatively structure information dissemination in order to stimulate patient partnership in decision making.

Lack of Perceived Consent

Lack of perceived consent illustrates another area of misunderstanding concerning malpractice. In acute care situations, patients may not perceive that they have really consented to a specific treatment even though all aspects of informed consent have been followed. If something upset them in retrospect, they may conclude that they were essentially coerced into what the physician suggested. Again, the importance of patients knowing about their own health problems and being aware of the specific problems that may arise is paramount to minimizing malpractice.

In summary, the malpractice situation could be improved if (1) patients know more about their own health; (2) patients know what to expect from providers so that they understand proposed care; (3) results are not unexpected; and (4) patients can become real partners in all decisions made. Achieving these improvements requires a system of providers who are much more proactive in educating, discussing and listening to patients (Hickson, et al., 1994). It also means that doctors working together decide as a group how they will treat common conditions and focus more on what they do as a group and less on what they do with each individual patient. For example, if a group of physicians is collaborating effectively, all members of the group should decide what position they will take on removing a particular organ. Then, patients will receive the same message from each physician and will not be confused. In addition, if there is legal action, the group can respond that it had adopted a specific clinical policy or protocol. They had *a priori* concluded that a specific approach was best for patients with a specific malady. Unless there is a cogent reason to change policy for a specific patient, the group's predetermined approach is to follow a specific protocol.

MINIMIZING MALPRACTICE THROUGH QUALITY IMPROVEMENT

Protocols for medical practice can be simpler and less complicated. This is really a matter of integrating quality assurance or quality improvement within clinical protocols. Classically, physicians have used the doctor-patient relationship as the cornerstone of practice. This resulted in the focus of care remaining unique for each specific patient. Obviously, doctors and patients are all unique; but medical conditions are generally not. If the perspective is changed, patients with similar conditions are then not viewed as unique with respect to problems or treatments. Patients with similar conditions can be grouped together, and groups of doctors who care for them can decide on a common approach. This results in patients knowing what to expect, how to quantify outcomes and which treatment produces the fewest problems. The goal of zero failures or defects is vastly different in many respects from the classical goal of best practice.

Medical groups that are committed to achieving fewer defects and enhanced quality control as a means for addressing malpractice litigation have several options, as depicted in Figure 6.2. First, medical groups should define a quality improvement goal(s). This may be articulated as the fewest failures or zero defects. Second, the groups should identify key quality assurance or continuous quality improvement strategies, many of which can be borrowed from corporate applications. Prevalent strategies adapted to the medical group context include setting achievable quality control goals for specific medical procedures, redesigning service delivery processes from the ground up to remove obstacles to quality, informing patients about

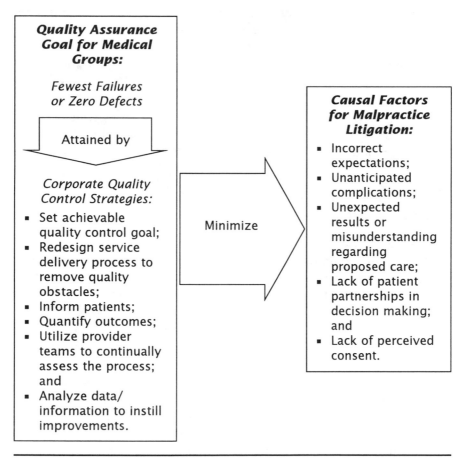

FIGURE 6.2   Quality Assurance as a Strategy to
Minimize Malpractice

the expectations associated with particular procedures, quantifying outcomes not only to track progress but also to aid in sharing information with patients, utilizing provider teams to continually assess the care delivery process and associated outcomes, and analyzing data/information to instill improvements. To the extent that medical groups adopt these and other quality control approaches borrowed from industry, it is feasible that the causal factors for malpractice litigation confronting medical groups can be reduced.

- An illustration may be helpful. Most would agree that there are a number of fine automobiles available to consumers at the present time. The prototype best car is well made, attractive, high-performing, of reasonable cost, and possesses a number of safety features to prevent accidents and to help save lives if there is an accident. If the ultimate goal for the best automobile was changed to ensure there would be no defects and no deaths from accidents, the cars would have to be quite different. One alternative is a car that could withstand a head-on collision at 40 miles per hour without passenger harm. It would be heavy and well armored. The top speed would be 20 miles per hour so that if two cars crashed head-on, their combined speed would not be above 40 miles per hour. The gas mileage might be 2 to 4 gallons per mile. This would create a quite different vehicle from the car we call best at the present time.

The previous illustration is extreme. If we are to move to a no-defects goal in medicine, the results would not be that bad. First, it would be necessary to change from an emphasis on process to an emphasis on an outcome goal. This has always been considered impossible in health care because every patient is unique. A large part of the rationale for staying with the process-based system is the fact that individual doctors are treating individual patients and each dyad is very different and possibly unique. In other words, each doctor-patient relationship represents a handmade, custom interaction with the diagnosis and treatment specifically made for that patient.

Before a high percentage of the population possessed insurance coverage, clinic services were provided in large hospitals and in some medical schools. In these clinics, treatment was not customized for individual patients. The patients were cared for by resident physicians in training, and the method of treatment for a certain diagnosis was decided by the chief of service. The clinics were considered a secondary class of service by most people, and there was a lack of privacy (due to teaching interventions) so that patients who could afford private care would not go to clinics. However, from an outcome results point of view, in many cases the results were better in the clinic than in the private service of the same hospital. Care delivery routines can be developed for certain symptoms and diagnoses that will provide exceptional results from an outcome point of view (that is, no defects).

To achieve the results, costs included, one must change the perspective of quality from process to outcome and utilize some of the lessons learned in business in this area. One of the best viewpoints is the six sigma concept adopted by Motorola and other enlightened corporations. **"Six sigma" is a term attached to the concept of achieving approximately zero defects in 3.4 million opportunities. The goal is to determine an ideal mean for the process and then have minimal standard deviation from the mean. The key to quality is to keep the variation as close to the mean as possible.**

To illustrate the enormity of the undertaking, the quality of most manufacturing processes in the United States is about three sigma, or 66,810 defects per million opportunities for error. Remember that six sigma is 3.4 defects per million opportunities for error. To begin to implement the goal of six sigma, the entire process of production or service delivery requires rethinking. One needs to start with a clean sheet of paper and design a new process. The standard process is examined, the mean is centered at an ideal point and the variation is reduced.

To begin this process in health care requires a shift in thinking. First, it is necessary to accept the fact that health care is comprised of a number of processes that can be standardized. Second, outcomes (not processes) must be articulated as a quality end point. Third, the variation in the process of delivering care must be reduced. This will be difficult in health care because most physicians have been, by experience, individually delivering one model of care. If two excellent physicians had the opportunity to deliver the same model of care, the results would be different. Moreover, by the nature of medical practice, physicians have tended to make the process more complex and unique rather than to simplify it. **For six sigma, each step in the process must be identified, considered in detail, simplified or omitted, and a new, less complex process developed. Then the new process is again examined to determine whether or not steps can be further simplified or omitted. Finally, the end process must be examined to see how crucial steps can be measured so that progress or lack thereof can be determined.**

REGULATION

Regulation in medical practice and health care has a rather long and convoluted history evolving from shortcomings in the delivery of care (Weil & Battistella, 1998). From the beginning, most medical regulations were procedural rather than outcome oriented. To satisfy the regulations, evidence of specific training (that is, a residency or preceptorship with the concept of time in training) was also important. For hospital privileges, doctors needed a year of internship or two to four years of residency. As time went on, individuals had to take and pass examinations at the end of training such as board exams in a specialty. In some instances, they had to submit a list of patients for whom they provided care along with a discussion of the results.

Over the years, regulations multiplied, but the background ideas are quite similar. Regulations to ensure quality are still procedurally oriented rather than outcome oriented. People have tried to find some way of using outcomes to evaluate care, but, because patients are seldom identical with exactly the same conditions, attempts at regulating via outcome are difficult, if not impossible. In the search for quality, continuing education has become a requirement for relicensure. To renew their licenses, physicians must take a certain number of courses normally delivered by medical school faculties. If a physician successfully completes a course, a certain number of points for each hour of the course are awarded. A specific number of points are required for relicensure.

The Joint Commission on Accreditation of Healthcare Organizations (JCAHO) has been the body charged with regulation of hospitals for the last 50 years. Its approach to licensing hospitals began as a logical implementation for the problems of that time. To receive accreditation, hospitals had to appoint committees to review practice. Tissue, infection control, operating room and mortality committees are several examples of mandated committees by the JCAHO. Committees would meet regularly and review the activities under their purview. The JCAHO also established goals for staff structure, clinical reviews and record maintenance.

A new thrust in quality control has been the adoption of care plans reflecting a standard of care. A group of involved doctors, nurses and administrators meet on a committee to develop a detailed care plan on how to treat a common entity (Smith, Yourstone, Lorber, & Mann, 2001). The goal is an agreed-upon standard of care for this entity that will be put into practice and utilized by the entire staff. The background for the care plan is that it should incorporate the highest-quality care.

Problems with Regulation as a Means to Control Quality

There are a number of problems with the regulatory approach to maintaining quality of care. The most serious problem is caused by the lack of results orientation in a regulatory approach. Today, very little medical care is provided by one person. Care is complex and the results are due to the effort of a group of individuals. An office visit amply illustrates this point. First, a receptionist has to provide a satisfactory appointment. The nurse has to meet the patient in the office and create some kind of bond that enables the patient to feel that there is caring and kindness. Then, the doctor has to diagnose and treat appropriately and effectively. Another person has to aid the patient with payment (for example, filling out forms). The outcome of that particular visit would not be satisfactory if anyone failed in his or her task or if the group did not function as a team. In large offices or hospitals, not functioning as a team is often the problem.

Procedural reviews in medical clinics may show that all staff are qualified and that each did his or her job well. Nonetheless, care may be negatively affected because there was no cooperation among group members. Rigorous reviews of results would document a problem immediately. But often the data are not available or the wrong data are reviewed. Hospitals have their own unique problems in reviewing performance. Mortality and morbidity reviews only show deaths and serious complications. The concept is that there should be no deaths and few serious complications. When deaths do occur, they are easily explained most of the time. The same is often true of serious complications. However, minor complications are not reviewed, and the individuals involved are virtually never flagged or recognized for their deficiencies. Nonetheless, here is where the majority of quality problems arise.

As in many other areas of quality control, regulations began to solve some real problems that were occurring at that time. However, due to enormous changes during the past decades, current methods of regulating medical care are expensive, cumbersome and ineffective.

Regulation has not provided the platform for addressing quality issues associated with the health care crisis.

LEGISLATION

A third retaliatory behavior that can result from poor-quality care is legislation. If enough patients suffer diminished outcomes due to problems in service delivery, it is possible that the political process will generate new laws governing the structure and process of care delivery. In turn, legislation prescribes an entire framework of regulations. Unlike malpractice litigation wherein an individual can initiate action in view of substandard care, regulation and legislation normally require a critical mass of public opinion in order to become reality. This relationship between regulation and legislation is depicted in Figure 6.3.

Consumer-Driven Revolution to Control Managed Care Failures

In 1996, 400 antimanaged care bills were proposed in states across the country; more than four times that in 1994 (American Association of Health Plans).

Examples of legislative issues:

- Physician "gag clauses" that prevent physicians from informing patients about treatment options;
- Maternity length of stay (>48 hours);
- Disclosure of physician incentives; and
- Provider network rules.

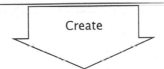

Create

Undesired Implications

- Heightened regulation
- The market is not functioning sufficiently to produce responsible health plans.

FIGURE 6.3   The Rise of Antimanaged Care Legislation

Managed care has gradually raised the threshold of pain for many consumers whether it is through decreased access to physicians, lowered amenity level in the receipt of care, exclusions on pharmaceutical use, earlier than desired hospital discharge or other undesirable effects. Consumers are quite simply angry about the treatment they feel they should be receiving when they are paying such enormous amounts of money in premiums. Consequently, in 1996, more than 400 antimanaged care bills were proposed in states across the country to try to alleviate at least some of the dysfunctions (Azevedo, 1996). This change represents a staggering four-fold increase over the number of bills introduced in 1994.

The antimanaged care legislation is focused on rectifying so-called physician "gag clauses," which HMOs have implemented to control what physicians share with patients about treatment options. It is also trying to ensure a minimum postpartum stay. Other popular bills have sought to force HMOs to disclose the system of physician incentives underlying a health plan so that patients have some insight as to why physicians recommend one course of action over another. Still other legislation has been directed toward clarifying rules that physicians are constrained by in networks.

The consumer-driven revolution to control managed care failures has been most successful in promoting a patient bill of rights that tempers HMO efforts to restrict patient services. In the end, this legislation creates undesired implications. More legislation drives more regulations and a bureaucracy to enforce the regulations. This ultimately costs both managed care plans and consumers more money. More legislation also indicates that the free market is inefficient—it is not functioning sufficiently to produce responsible health plans.

In the end, increased legislation, like regulation, is an unfortunate by-product of poor-quality health care. It constrains both provider and consumer alike. A far better alternative is for quality care to surround service delivery.

The context of health care is vividly affected by trends in legislation leading to new policies regarding medical payment, regulations and liabilities. Fee-for-service medicine lasted for decades and created a system of perquisites and cost structure that are now difficult to reverse. Although managed care and capitated payment have surfaced as mechanisms to control payment malfunctions, these control mechanisms are having to address an enormous base and years of inflationary increases. Regulation has been both a control on and a contributor to the health crisis. Care standards and professional control have hampered efforts to instill incentives and open the system to competitive forces. However, regulation has also promoted high-quality care delivery and prevented excessive hospital construction. Malpractice has driven up costs, encouraged duplication and generated defensive medicine because of the ease in suing medical providers.

While these factors underlying the health crisis represent the foundation for health care redesign, they also offer a path for medical groups that are intent on transcending the quagmire. Medical groups can benefit substantially in their own reconstruction efforts by addressing legislation, regulation and malpractice in nontraditional ways. Perhaps a group will capitalize on the pressure of malpractice liability to forge a new set of physician or provider relations with patients, recognizing that most malpractice is avoidable through care delivery strategies that enhance the experience for providers as well. Alternatively, a group may rethink its thrust to assemble an integrated set of clinics, recognizing that growth for the sake of bargaining power with managed care plans effectively undermines the group's ability to maintain focus and inordinately high quality—two superior bargaining chips in the tumultuous health care arena.

In short, the analysis of malpractice litigation, regulation and legislation provides more than a base for understanding the antecedents to health care reform. The analysis is more than just a descriptive examination of factors that have escalated in producing a stranglehold over health care delivery. It is a scorecard against which physicians and medical groups can assess the efficacy of their efforts to build strategies consistent with high performance.

QUALITY CARE THROUGH BUSINESS PRACTICES AND CONTINUOUS IMPROVEMENT

The potential threats of malpractice litigation, regulation and liability should be incentive enough for health care providers to maintain a consistent vigilance on the quality of service delivery. However, what is quality? What are the exact dimensions or attributes that form quality of care? Once a definition of quality has been reached, what strategies can physicians and medical groups use to improve service delivery and the outcomes associated with service delivery? Answers to these questions surface from an extensive literature on quality of care derived from applied research in medicine and health. Promising answers are also found in the business setting where total quality management and continuous quality improvement have revolutionized how businesses deliver services and produce goods.

The Elusive Definition of Quality

The starting point in any quality assurance or quality improvement process is to initially define the term "quality." Such a definition is elusive, a fact that has hounded practitioners and researchers for years. Part of the consternation involves the theoretical and practical differences between service quality and customer satisfaction (Taylor, 1994). It has been argued that service quality and consumer satisfaction are entirely separate constructs (Parasuraman, Zeithaml, & Berry, 1985) that, although similar in nature, really speak to different organizational objectives. Other authorities express the belief that service quality and customer satisfaction are closely related and strongly correlated, thus justifying the view that they are equivalent constructs (Bowers, Swan, & Koehler, 1994; Woodside, Lisa, & Daly, 1989).

In developing survey instrumentation to measure service quality, emphasis has focused on specifying the explicit dimensions, or attributes, that capture quality outcomes. Following are three representative examples of service quality dimensions:

Jun, Peterson & Zsidisin (1998)	Parasuraman, Zeithaml & Berry (1985)	Bowers, Swan & Koehler (1994)
Tangibles	Tangibles	Tangibles
Realiability	Realiability	Realiability
Responsiveness	Responsiveness	Responsiveness
Competence	Competence	Competence
Courtesy	Courtesy	Courtesy
Communication	Communication	Communication
Access	Credibility	Credibility
Caring	Security	Security
Patient Outcomes	Access	Access
Understanding Patient	Understanding Customer	Understanding Patient
Collaboration		Caring
		Patient Outcomes

Tangibles generally refer to the appearance or cleanliness of a health facility (or staff members). For further insights on the specific attributes comprising the dimensions of quality, see Sidebar 6.2.

SIDEBAR 6.2

Quality Dimensions in Health Care

Jun, Peterson and Zsidisin (1998) conducted focus group interviews in a public, mid-sized hospital serving a community of approximately 70,000 people in the Southwest as a means of clarifying the dimensions of service quality. Three focus groups were formed. First, an interview group was formed of six middle-level administrative staffers including vice presidents for human resources, nursing and planning among other managerial positions. Second, a focus group was formed using six patients, several of whom were employed at the hospital. Third, the final group was comprised of four resident physicians who staff the family practice facility at the hospital. The obvious strength of this study is the effort to include several constituents in the specification of service quality dimensions. Balanced against this strength is the relatively limited sample size of individuals providing insights on service quality. Therefore, the results of this study should be interpreted cautiously. Nonetheless, the findings generally corroborate previous studies about service quality dimensions.

The focus group interviews identified the following dimensions:

1. Tangibles associated with service delivery:
   - Appearance;
   - Processes; and
   - Cleanliness.
2. Courtesy of providers and staff:
   - Attitude;
   - Privacy; and
   - Professionalism.
3. Reliability of service delivery:
   - Consistency (that is, equal treatment); and
   - Billing accuracy.
4. Communication with providers and staff:
   - Technical complexity explained;
   - Sufficient interaction; and
   - Amount of time spent with specific providers.
5. Competence displayed or suggested by providers and staff:
   - Education;

continued

- Expected; and
- Continual improvement.

6. Understanding the customer:
   - Patient; and
   - Physician.

7. Access:
   - Visibility; and
   - Convenience.

8. Responsiveness

9. Caring

10. Patient outcomes

11. Collaboration:
    - Teamwork;
    - Synergistic package; and
    - Internal and external to hospital.

It is interesting to note that a dimension of "patient outcomes" was indicated by the focus groups to represent a specific dimension of service quality. There have been mixed recommendations regarding whether outcomes should be regarded as a separate dimension of quality compared to the other perceptual dimensions.

Although the administrators, patients and physicians generally agreed on the dimensions comprising health care quality, a number of important differences surfaced in the course of the interviews, as follows:

	Administrators	*Patients*	*Physicians*
1. Tangibles	+	+	+*
2. Courtesy	+	+	NM†
3. Reliability	+	+	+
4. Communication	+	+	+
5. Competence	+	+	+
6. Understanding Patient	+	+	+
7. Access	+	+	+
8. Responsiveness	+	+	-‡
9. Caring	NM	+	-
10. Patient Outcomes	+	NM	+
11. Collaboration	+	+	+

Note: *Important dimension; †not mentioned; ‡not important or negative connotation

continued

Administrators did not mention "caring" as an important service dimension. Physicians did not mention "courtesy" as a key dimension. Patients did not discuss "outcomes" as an important, perceived dimension of service quality. In many respects, these omissions fit precisely with stereotypical views of providers and customers. Administrators are most concerned with delivering a product or service without addressing the emotional or feeling aspects of delivery. Physicians are focused on the technical aspects of care and, thus, are not entirely cognizant of the importance of courtesy. Patients want a comfortable experience regardless of the outcome from service delivery. Again, caution should be used in interpreting the results of this study, but the findings do give physicians and medical groups food for thought about their predispositions and the importance of recalibrating professional attitudes that can adversely influence patient perceptions of service quality.

Source: Adapted from M. Jun, R. T. Peterson, & G. A. Zsidisin. (1998). The identification and measurement of quality dimensions in health care: Focus group interview results. *Health Care Management Review, 23*(4), 81–96.

It is appropriate to consider the Joint Commission on Accreditation of Healthcare Organizations (1996), which has identified nine quality dimensions:

Dimension	*Definition*
Efficacy	• Efficacy of the procedure or treatment in relation to the patient's condition • The degree to which the care of the patient has been shown to accomplish the desired or projected outcome(s)
Appropriateness	• Appropriateness of a specific test, procedure or service to meet the patient's needs • The degree to which the care provided is relevant to the patient's clinical needs, given the current state of knowledge
Ffficiency	• Efficiency with which services are provided • The relationship between the outcomes (results of care) and the resources used to deliver patient care
Respect and Caring	• Respect and caring with which services are provided • The degree to which the patient or a designee is involved in his or her own care decisions and to which those providing services do so with sensitivity and respect for the patient's needs, expectations and individual differences

Safety	• Safety of the patient (and others) to whom the services are provided
	• The degree to which the risk of an intervention and risk in the care environment are reduced for the patient and others, including the health care provider
Continuity	• Continuity of the services provided to the patient with respect to other services, practitioners and providers and over time
	• The degree to which the care for the patient is coordinated among practitioners, among organizations, and over time
Effectiveness	• Effectiveness with which tests, procedures, treatments and services are provided
	• The degree to which the care is provided in the correct manner, given the current state of knowledge, to achieve the desired or projected outcome for the patient
Timeliness	• Timeliness with which a needed test, procedure, treatment or service is provided to the patient
	• The degree to which the care is provided to the patient at the most beneficial or necessary time
Availability	• Availability of a needed test, procedure, treatment or service to the patient who needs it
	• The degree to which appropriate care is available to meet the patient's needs

As the Joint Commission quality dimensions suggest, quality is multidimensional. Therefore, a single definition of quality care will be difficult to reach in many care delivery settings. For physicians and medical groups, the issue is not so much which is the correct definition, but rather that analysis and discussion have preceded the selection of dimensions that will guide service delivery.

The preceding discussion of quality dimensions underscores the reality that despite significant interest in defining what constitutes quality, the health care field has distinct problems in arriving at a single, acceptable definition. Quality varies by setting whether it is for hospital accreditation, physician or nurse licensure or medical group performance. As one physician has described quality:

> No one knows how to properly measure it or who is accountable for it, but everyone knows it should be maximized, risk-adjusted, reported to the public and of low cost. Plans should compete on it, and physicians should be judged on it (La Puma, 1998).

Thus, quality care is an elusive concept yet one that no provider can overlook or minimize in efforts to deliver services.

Despite the obvious admonition that all providers should upgrade their efforts at attaining quality, it is valuable to pause and reflect on this charge, particularly in view of the vagaries surrounding the concept of quality. Is quality improvement attainable in a managed care environment where cost-control policies and practices have threatened even the ability to deliver basic services? This is a serious question, yet one that is constantly in mind when physicians attempt to deliver care.

Manian (1998) captures the sense of alienation and loss of control that many practitioners experience in an essay on how managed care is driving medical practice to mediocrity. Manian documents the many deficiencies, errors and frustrations that characterize care delivery today. Several examples are shown in Table 6.1.

Manian's illustrations suggest that quality of care will continue to be elusive as long as cost control erodes the very basis for acceptable or satisfactory care delivery. In other words, it is difficult to even think of quality improvement when the current delivery system is constantly eroding. Mediocrity has become acceptable and the standard for quality of care reduced. Undoubtedly, many of Manian's physician colleagues will resonate with the examples displayed in Table 6.1. Nonetheless, the situation may not be as dismal as Manian portrays. Physicians still exercise great control over medical practice, and health care organizations recognize that quality of care is a tangible outcome that retains and attracts patients (and patient groups). Manian also overlooks the fact that new and innovative processes are surfacing in medical practice and administration that offer optimism for improving quality of care in the future.

Continuous Quality Improvement

Corporations have embraced many processes for instilling improvement, operating efficiently and raising quality (Heskett, Sasser, & Schlesinger, 1997). Whether total quality management, continuous quality improvement or reengineering, the goal remains the same—to produce better outcomes in the form of services and products. Philosophically, the efforts to improve business practices and outcomes are similar, even though they may utilize different tactics for achieving improvement. It is through these methodologies that

---

TABLE **6.1** Mediocrity in Medical Practice?

Farrin A. Manian argues against the ability of physicians to embrace quality improvement techniques due to the erosion of practice support. He does not argue against quality—only the efficacy of quality improvement programs in view of the economic changes that are constraining care. Following are several examples of what otherwise might appear to be minor deficiencies, errors and frustrations (DEFs). Manian's point is that these seemingly insignificant constraints accumulate. The sum effect is insidious for achieving quality of care.

DEF 1

Often my orders for laboratory tests on inpatients and outpatients are not carried out properly, resulting in the patients' having to undergo repeated phlebotomy and in delays in the reporting of important laboratory results.

The Problem: Those who are in charge of processing physicians' orders are hurried, do not have sufficient familiarity with the type of tests ordered because the job is not taken seriously by their employers (i.e., it is a relatively low paying job), have a short attention span, do not have enough common sense to ask for help when they need it, or have any combination of these traits.

DEF 3

Important information such as vital signs, medications, and status of the intravenous site is no longer predictably documented in the patients' charts, often necessitating the initiation of a fact-finding mission and interviews with the nursing staff before I can be reasonably certain what really happened.

The Problem: Members of the nursing staff are hurried, are not sufficiently trained, do not appreciate the importance of documenting patients' basic medical information in the chart, are so disgruntled that they don't care, or have any combination of these traits.

DEF 5

Changes in patients' clinical status (e.g., new onset of chills or changes in mental status) are not necessarily recognized by the nurse's assistants (at some places they are referred to as "patient care associates"), nor are additional vital signs measured, resulting in a delay in diagnosis and in the initiation of appropriate therapy.

The Problem: Those who hire non-nurse patient care workers to do nurses' jobs at lower wages seem to have underestimated the importance of the basic nursing skills required for recognizing when something is wrong. These skills cannot be acquired overnight, and yet miraculously anyone interested in taking vital

---

TABLE 6.1 Continued

signs and working in the health care field seems to have become qualified. Never mind that errors in the initial assessment of a patient's condition may have grave consequences for the overall quality of care, no matter how skillful or astute the clinician or the nurse in charge may be. Cost has to be kept down.

DEF 10

I often have to search in several places to find blank progress-note sheets (to write my daily progress notes in hospitalized patients' medical records), tongue blades, sterile swabs, and other supplies.

The Problem: Nobody assumes responsibility for having commonly used supplies where they should be—that is, next to the patients' rooms. The clerks are too busy placing the wrong orders in the computer. Are hospitals becoming self-serve, or should we ask physicians to adopt a BYOS (Bring Your Own Supplies) policy? By the way, what about my own efficiency when I can't find what I need to take care of patients? Is it not likely that if I constantly have to look for supplies, I will have less time to do what I am supposed to do in the first place, such as interviewing and examining patients, talking to their relatives, and reviewing laboratory reports?

Source: Adapted from F. A. Manian. (1998, April 19). Should we accept mediocrity? *New England Journal of Medicine, 338*(15), 1067–1069.

---

emphasize quality improvement that corporations in the United States have regained strength and the ability to compete globally.

In view of the widespread success of continuous improvement technologies, it would seem natural that the health and medical fields would enthusiastically embrace these practices. After all, many U.S. corporations were able to turn around their competitive capabilities and thrive in the global marketplace. Despite the many testimonials about the benefits of continuous improvement strategies, health care has been slow to adopt these programs. Arndt and Bigelow (1998) argue that the problem may be related to management fads and the lack of long-term legitimacy for temporal management techniques. Usually, these management fads lack proof of demonstrable, long-term results that convince skeptical personnel. In medicine, many physicians are inherently suspicious of management jargon and concepts that seem to lack depth. Accustomed to making medical decisions independently, many physicians see limited value in the consensus-based techniques of quality improvement. Unfortunately, it is precisely the magnitude of the health care crisis that implores the health care field to adopt new ways of delivering care.

The health care crisis offers a rich environment for the new management technologies. In particular, the health system needs both innovation and quality emphasis. Reengineering is "...the fundamental rethinking and radical redesign of business process to achieve dramatic improvement in critical, contemporary measures of performance, such as cost, quality, services, and speed" (Hammer & Champy, 1993, p. 332). Continuous quality improvement is the systematic analysis and improvement of production and service delivery. The key here is not the jargon, or the specific techniques attached to each program, but rather the concept that production/service delivery can be continuously improved in innovative ways and that the outcomes of production/service delivery can be successively improved.

Sidebar 6.3 reports details on a study of U.S. and Canadian hospitals that underscores the difficult progress of reengineering concepts. A sizable percentage of the respondents had never heard of reengineering. If substantial numbers of hospital executives are not familiar with reengineering, then it is plausible that physicians are also not aware of reengineering or its promise. Yet, hospitals that do adopt reengineering practices have in mind the improvement of (Ho, Chan, & Kidwell, 1999):

- Service quality to external customers;
- Financial performance;
- Clinical performance;
- Service quality to internal customers; and
- Processing time of service delivery.

To a lesser extent, hospitals report adopting reengineering programs to benefit like other health care organizations, to comply with regulations, to competitively stay in the game or to follow advice from a consultant.

Continuous quality improvement programs utilize six- to eight-member teams to identify and resolve problems. Participants are typically provided instruction in continuous improvement concepts and applications. Team leaders usually receive additional training in their

SIDEBAR 6.3

A Scorecard on Reengineering Applications in Hospitals

Ho, Chan and Kidwell (1999) studied the implementation of business process reengineering in 95 U.S. and 121 Canadian hospitals. Of the total hospitals responding to this survey, 17 percent indicated that they have never heard of business process reengineering. This is a depressing finding in view of the role that reengineering has played globally in the business sector. Seventy-four percent of those hospitals that have heard of reengineering have been implementing the process for more than one year, with 50 percent of the hospitals using the process on more than six projects.

Hospital executives indicated that the reengineering efforts have been most successful in:

- Improving financial performance;
- Improving clinical performance;
- Improving service quality to internal customers;
- Improving service quality to external customers (patients); and
- Improving processing time of service delivery.

The reengineering efforts were rated, on average, as moderately successful in accomplishing the desired objectives.

The Ho, Chan and Kidwell study is particularly useful in the medical field because it identified the factors that prevent successful business process reengineering:

- Lack of cooperation from staff as process reengineering is viewed as job cutting;
- Lack of buy-in from medical staff;
- Insufficient staff training and skill development on process reengineering;
- Poor planning;
- Lack of enthusiasm and interest;
- Insufficient staffing;
- Lack of access to information (for example, benchmarking data);
- Lack of funding;

- Too time-consuming to implement the reengineered process;
- Lack of support from labor union;
- No top-management support;
- Low priority;
- Too time-consuming to select and train employees;
- Internal control is not well defined under the new process reengineering project; and
- Personnel turnover

It is notable that 47 percent of the preceding factors were rated as contributing to some extent to the unsuccessful business process reengineering. The findings clearly indicate the importance of solid preparation of staff beforehand and incorporation of physician leaders to integrate medical staff cooperation.

Source: S. J. Ho, L. Chan, & R. E. Kidwell, Jr. (1999, Spring). The implementation of business process reengineering in American and Canadian hospitals. *Health Care Management Review, 24*(2), 19–31.

---

role as facilitators. The teams are data-driven; that is, they use surveys and performance reports (as well as knowledge of team participants) to identify problems and focus on an agenda for problem solving. The key operating rule for the team is consensus-based decision making. Authority does not dominate. The teams generally meet on a scheduled basis, but additional meetings are possible when addressing a particularly controversial issue in problem identification or resolution. Each team reports to a general council that oversees the quality improvement efforts.

The Milwaukee Medical Clinic is one example of a medical group that has adopted continuous quality improvement methodologies (Chesanow, 1997). The clinic is a multispecialty practice with more than 100 physicians and 750 employees delivering care at seven sites. Four steps comprise the clinic's improvement process:

Step 1:   **Problem identification**—A flowchart is created to analyze and identify problems. This visualization of the process often uncovers obvious glitches that can be resolved.

Step 2:   **Problem focus**—Data are collected to provide insights and confirm the identified problem. Visualization remains a key facilitating factor; consequently, data are prepared in charts, tables and other easy-to-interpret formats.

Step 3:   **Solution design**—The teams methodically suggest process improvements. A free-flowing dialogue with all team members participating is the ideal that team leaders strive to achieve. In many care delivery situations, the practice variations are detailed and the best practice is adopted.

Step 4:   **Implementation**—The best practice is implemented and monitored to verify that it delivers the anticipated results.

Specific results from Milwaukee Medical Clinic's continuous quality improvement process are reported in Sidebar 6.4. It is important to note that the biggest hindering factor has been physicians who are reluctant to accept group-based solutions.

The Milwaukee Medical Clinic is not the only health care provider that has reported success with continuous quality improvement and reengineering techniques. Whether seeking patient satisfaction (Gustafson & Hundt, 1995; Mack, File, Horwitz, & Prince, 1995) in medical settings or mental health settings (Ingram & Chung, 1997), quality im **In order for success to continue to occur, it is clear that top management, especially physician executives, must stand firmly behind the adoption and maintenance of reengineering and continuous quality improvement programs** (Yasin, Czuchry, Jennings, & York, 1999).

QUALITY CARE THROUGH CLINICAL AND OUTCOMES DATA

Spragins (1999) has made the case that health maintenance organizations are getting more secretive about their quality outcomes performance. If consumers are unable to access information on quality performance, then it will be difficult for them to compare one managed care plan's performance against another. In effect, they will lack the requisite information needed to make wise purchasing decisions. The National Committee for Quality Assurance (NCQA), a quasi-independent organization, sets accrediting standards for managed care plans. The NCQA assesses managed care plan quality performance through a set of 20 quality measures that form a Quality Compass. Spragins argues that increasingly, managed care plans are not permit-

SIDEBAR 6.4
Continuous Quality Improvement Victories

When the multispecialty Milwaukee Medical Clinic adopted continuous quality improvement methodologies to improve services and outcomes, it had little idea that the process would be so successful. Following are several examples of victories that surfaced in the use of continuous improvement techniques:

Radiology-Reports Team:

Problem: MMC's X-ray staff didn't know where to send the physician copy of an X-ray report, especially if the doctor worked in several MMC satellite locations.

Solution: A new protocol was designed: When physicians request an X-ray, they use the radiology department's computer system to indicate where the copy should be sent. The location thus appears on the printed radiology report, eliminating guesswork by X-ray personnel.

Rehab Authorization/Managed-Care Team:

Problem: The time it took to receive an authorization for rehab care from insurance companies seemed overly long.

Solution: MMC's managed care department and rehab manager, along with insurance company representatives, identified clinical information that MMC was neglecting to send to insurers. Therapists were made aware that insurance coverage for therapy wasn't all-inclusive, and they were taught how to document information the insurance companies required. The rehab procedure was redesigned to guarantee that no more than two patient visits were permitted prior to an insurance company authorization. Patients also now receive a form stating that their insurance may not cover all rehab services, reducing misunderstandings.

Documentation Team:

Problem: The transcription department was spending significant time trying to figure out whether physicians' dictation was completed, or whether handwritten notes were supposed to accompany the transcription tape. In addition, about 18 percent of all transcribed chart notes contained errors or were incomplete, resulting in documents that were unprofessional and potentially litigious.

continued

Solution: Doctors were given codes to indicate whether their notes were dictated or handwritten. An often-ignored policy that doctors' notes are to be dictated with 24 hours and transcribed within 72 hours of seeing a patient was given new force. A doctor who doesn't provide timely dictation is notified by the transcription department.

Lab/Oncology Team:

Problem: Sending specimens from the oncology department to the pathology lab, processing and testing the specimens and relaying the results to MMC oncologists took too long.

Solution: Installing an inexpensive light system with an audible alarm to alert the lab to a specimen delivery alleviated the phone traffic that was a substantial cause of the problem. Changes in the lab's hematology department cut turnaround time on key tests to 10 minutes. Test-ordering procedures were changed to improve communication among reception, the oncology department and the pathology lab.

Walk-in Services Team:

Problem: Progress notes on patients seen in walk-in service's were not readily available for follow-up. When these patients called their primary doctors for test results or to ask questions about their treatment, the notes had not been entered on their charts.

Solution: The medical records department now gives priority to walk-in service's progress notes, reducing the filing time from 10 days to 2, on average. A pediatric phone nurse, who assumed responsibility for contacting parents of pediatric walk-in patients, receives the progress notes from walk-in services and phones parents the next day. Previously, parents waited four days to get a call.

Pharmacy Team:

Problem: The distribution of pharmaceutical supplies to various departments and clinic satellites needed to be improved. Written orders were often illegible, frequent phone orders were too time-consuming for pharmacists to field, deliveries were late, some items were outdated, and there was no uniform stock requisition form.

Solution: The team drafted procedures for ordering supplies, filling and billing pharmacy orders, and delivering supplies to MMC satellites. A computer database of all pharmacy supplies was compiled for easy access. And a new pharmacy stock order sheet, customized for each department's needs, was developed.

The biggest constraint on success of the continuous improvement approach has been reluctance on the part of physicians to participate. This is understandable because most physicians have been trained to accumulate knowledge before making decisions. Continuous improvement methodologies require a team-based approach wherein decision making is shared among many types of professionals and nonprofessionals. Naturally, physicians have a difficult time accepting group decision making and shared authority.

Source: Adapted from N. Chesanow. (1997, August 11). Making doctors' lives easier-and patients happier. *Medical Economics*, 119–131.

---

ting the NCQA to release their performance on the Quality Compass. Without a consistent set of comparable standards that the Quality Compass represents, consumers lack benchmark performance data and, thus, are ill-equipped to make intelligent purchase decisions.

Spragins recommends that consumers petition their company's benefits office to provide Quality Compass data for shopping comparisons. This consumer advocacy approach demonstrates the direction that the health care field is taking toward disclosure and outcome benchmarking. The problem for health care has been identifying a set of quality performance measures that have the backing of providers (Landon, Wilson, & Cleary, 1998). The NCQA has usurped the formation of these standards by the medical community ostensibly because physicians have fought tenaciously against outcomes standards and practice guidelines. The NCQA bases its Quality Compass on benchmarks derived from the Health Plan Employer Data and Information Set (HEDIS). HEDIS measures are not entirely untainted, as progressive refinements in measures of care occur each year (Kuttner, 1998). Thus, a measure of diabetes care activity and outcomes may not be the same from year to year, which aggravates the ability to make valid comparisons.

The significant implication from NCQA, Quality Compass and HEDIS is that medical groups and physicians will increasingly be called on to document their care delivery quality (and performance). Orlando (1998) indicates that physicians and medical groups can anticipate requests for patient-oriented, patient-centered and patient-reported data. In short, providers will need the backing of clinical information systems that document clinical information (that is, clinical practice activity) and outcomes from care delivery. This will require substantial investment in electronic record keeping and in broader clinical information systems that support decisions and reporting (Murray, 1996).

Information becomes the driver for continuous quality improvement of clinical practice. Pizzo (1995) recommends that physicians build quality improvement upon diverse sets of information. Hard evidence through data becomes a means for physicians to prove to health plans the quality of care that they deliver. Pizzo specifically suggests:

1. Identifying and tracking a physician's most common diagnoses to monitor revenue per diagnosis, frequency of hospitalization and mortality statistics;

2. Comparing average length of stay, utilization rate by diagnosis and cost per admission with colleagues; and

3. Building practice guidelines and treatment protocols to stabilize and instill consistency in care delivery.

In short, information becomes the basis for continuous quality improvement whether in a private clinic or large group practice.

The trends in data reporting and continuous quality improvement suggest that physicians and medical groups should contemplate robust clinical information systems. In this regard, the formation and evolution of clinical information will be diverse and inclusive of a wide variety of performance areas. Consumers assess quality of care along many dimensions beyond quality, as shown in Sidebar 6.5. As the health care system becomes increasingly competitive, physicians and medical groups can use data to improve their operations and then to convey to many stakeholders the efficacy of their efforts.

Medical groups that aspire to deliver the right care at the right time with kindness and low cost face the imperative of proving that they can deliver the goods. It is one thing to aspire to a lofty goal and quite another to verify the integrity of service delivery and the ability to achieve diverse objectives. Quality of care is an elusive goal that is difficult to measure just as it is difficult to measure low-cost care (Waress, Pasternak, & Smith, 1994), kind care or timeliness of care (Dixon & Trenchard, 1996). Clinical data and quality outcome data are only one portion of a systematic and comprehensive performance assessment capability that medical groups must develop if they expect to be delivering care in the future.

SIDEBAR 6.5

Hospital Shopping by a Rural Community

Most health care authorities would argue that the quality of care is the primary consideration that patients use in deciding to receive services from a provider. Their argument may be incorrect. Taylor and Capella (1996) investigated the attributes used by citizens in a rural community of 36,000 people in selecting a hospital for inpatient treatment. The population has essentially two choices for acute care services: They can either receive care from a local hospital or they can seek care from competitors in other communities, particularly a major metropolitan area 45 miles away. A total of 410 households participated in the project. In order to be included in the sample, someone in the household must have received medical services from a hospital within the last three years.

What are the criteria by which the respondents choose a hospital to receive care? Quality of care was not the most important determinant, although quality of hospital services was ranked among the top four selection criteria:

Criteria	Rank
Convenient location	1
Modern facility	2
Good appearance of rooms	3
Quality of hospital services	4
Overall appearance of hospital	5
Quality of hospital facility	6
Good reputation	7
Courtesy/friendliness of employees	8
Modern equipment/technology	9
Quality of hospital personnel	10
Full range of services	11
Specialty physicians on staff	12
Quality of physicians	13
Quality of nursing care	14
Competitive costs of services	15

It is interesting to observe that quality of physician services and quality of nursing services were ranked very low by the residents in terms of their importance in selecting a hospital. This is surprising for nursing care because nursing care is such an important part of hospital services.

In contrast, the ratings for quality of physician services might be ranked much higher if the residents were asked to rate the determinants of their choice for physician care.

Further insights on hospital choice surfaced when Taylor and Capella compared determinants for those who received care at the local community hospital versus those who received care from a hospital outside the community:

Outshoppers		Inshoppers	
Criteria	*Rank*	*Criteria*	*Rank*
Convenient location	1	Convenient location	1
Competitive costs of services	2	Quality of hospital services	2
Quality of hospital facility	3	Good reputation	3
Overall appearance of hospital	4	Modern facility	4
Good appearance of rooms	5	Courtesy/friendliness of employees	5
Modern facility	6	Quality of hospital personnel	6
Full range of services	7	Good appearance of rooms	7
Modern equipment/technology	8	Overall appearance of hospital	8
Specialty physicians on staff	9	Modern equipment/ technology	9
Quality of hospital personnel	10	Quality of hospital facility	10
Courtesy/friendliness of employees	11	Full range of services	11
Quality of nursing care	12	Quality of physicians	12
Quality of hospital services	13	Specialty physicians on staff	13
Quality of physicians	14	Quality of nursing care	14
Good reputation	15	Competitive costs of services	15
Grand mean = .989		Grand mean = 1.194	

Those who receive care outside the community (outshoppers) considered factors such as convenient location, cost, facility quality, and appearance of the hospital and its rooms. The lowest-rated determinants were quality of nursing care, hospital services and physicians, as well as a good reputation for the hospital they selected. Thus, quality of care appears not to be a significant determinant for those residents who went outside the community for hospital care. This finding seems to be counterintuitive; we would expect those selecting hospital care outside the community to be seeking higher quality of care. Further, it is paradoxical that local residents who seek care at hospitals outside the community do so because of the convenient location of those other facilities.

Those residents who elected to receive care at the local hospital expressed similar confounding results. As anticipated, they ranked convenient location as the primary determinant for receiving care at the local facility. However, the second most important factor for selecting the local hospital is quality of the hospital services. These residents clearly believe that their local hospital is capable of delivering high quality of care. Of course, the unanswered question is, does the local hospital really deliver high-quality care? This question was not answered in the study by Taylor and Capella. In the same vein, it is not clear that the residents have solid knowledge about why they rate the local hospital so highly on quality of services.

Source: Adapted from: S. L. Taylor & L. M. Capella. (1996). Hospital outshopping: Determinant attributes and hospital choice. *Health Care Management Review, 21*(4), 33–44.

APPLICATIONS FOR MANAGERS

Every medical clinic and provider needs an active program to ensure high performance in delivering quality care. Quality always sells; low cost is popular but seldom in a trade-off with quality when it comes to health care products and services. Medical providers normally focus on addressing the points at which they are vulnerable for malpractice litigation, but this approach falls far short of what it takes to become a high-performing entity. All staff should want to meet the standards for exemplary care; but for a medical clinic seeking to establish itself as a leader, staff should also aspire to greatly exceed those standards.

The first step for medical practice executives is establishing a base for assuring quality and minimizing potential litigation. Managers should focus their attention on several key areas.

1. Working with clinical providers to devise programs for better informing patients about expectations for care—Clinicians have the best chance of helping patients understand what to expect in the way of the course of treatment, the probabilities for unexpected results, specific actions that must be taken in the event of complications, indicators of complications; steps for recovery and what to do for follow-up. However, managers should also cultivate staff to help reinforce clinical education and instruction and to provide multiple avenues for identifying and resolving problems before they occur. The goal is to have duplicate systems to ensure quality without duplicating cost.

2. Establishing systems to address complications—After clinicians and staff inform patients about the potential for complications, there remains the challenge of creating systems to alleviate unanticipated problems. Most medical groups assume that clinicians will simply handle the matter as a course of treatment. However, think of the potential for building quality that might result from having a special case manager to follow up on all patients when problems arise. This tactic would help to improve patient satisfaction with care. It would facilitate getting the right care at the right time to the patient. It would also establish a monitoring system to support efforts at continuous quality improvement. Of course, the immediate concern of most clinic managers is who will pay for this service. It is quite likely that the costs of a dedicated nurse would be offset by greater efficiency in care delivery (that is, less disruption of ongoing care delivery by physicians and other medical team members) and by greater cooperation (and satisfaction) of patients.

3. Building patient understanding about proposed care—Although physicians tend to resist using clinical practice guidelines or protocols, medical practice executives should work to encourage the use of published protocols in educating patients. Physicians have to recognize that patients only hear part of the instructions and explanation that are intended for them. By having written protocols (derived from the more technical and clinically sophisticated protocols used by medical staff) available for dissemination to patients, it is possible to greatly enhance understanding about proposed care.

4. Incorporating patients in care decisions—Once patients have been fully informed (preferably through presentation of written protocols and expectations), it is appropriate to establish their participation in the care process. A contract for care would spell out precisely what actions the patient is responsible for before and after treatment. These contracts would be developed in concert with the clinical protocol which spells out expectations for the structure and process of care.

5. Attaining complete patient consent—If providers have carefully explained the structure and process for care, detailed the possibilities and probabilities for complications and explained the responsibilities for patients, then patients are better prepared to join in the decision and to consent to care delivery. Medical practice executives can create informed consent by building the basics of education and information surrounding care delivery mentioned in the preceding four points.

Another valuable strategy for ensuring high performance in care delivery and preventing malpractice litigation is to design and implement continuous quality improvement programs. Managed care plans and accredited providers are required in a regulatory sense to maintain such programs. Quality sells. It demonstrates a tangible and distinctive difference in a product or service. Therefore, quality also has tremendous value to the medical group that is able to deliver the outcome.

For those medical groups that do not have systematic and comprehensive quality assurance and improvement programs, the message is clear. Develop quality review efforts in order to create a more valuable service for patients and insurers—this is a fundamental key to long-run success. For the majority of medical groups that already have ongoing quality management programs, the message is equally clear. Ratchet your program up another notch or level. Evidence-based or outcome-based medicine is acknowledged as the future for medical practice. The concept should be extrapolated to all aspects of clinical services, including administration.

Medical groups can profit considerably by conducting discussions about what constitutes quality service delivery among all staff. For example, multidisciplinary provider teams may discover that the root of their problems in building better quality centers on differences of opinion about what quality are consists of how patients perceive service delivery. In another case, housekeeping and maintenance may learn that their definition of quality differs substantially from that conceived by the nursing staff. The point is to introduce a broader spectrum of information considered in continuous quality improvement processes. Discussion creates the basis for understanding and subsequent refinement of service delivery processes.

Medical practice executives can also improve their quality improvement programs by seeking the best practice data and performance benchmarks. One option may be creating a strategic alliance with five other medical groups in a specific geographical location to define patient satisfaction with clinical care. Members in the group alliance might agree to use the same postvisit survey as a means to generate benchmarks for comparative purposes. In other cases, clinic managers will seek state- and national-level data from professional associations. Internal benchmarks are always useful, but there is nothing like external comparisons to provide insight on possibilities for improvement.

In the final analysis, medical practice executives face a difficult problem in implementing continuous quality improvement. No one pays for continuous improvement, except indirectly. Physicians and nurses are already overburdened with providing care and have little interest in looking back—they are focusing on the present. Despite these obstacles, there is an imperative to build even stronger and far-reaching programs at assuring quality and efficacious resource use. Medical groups that will be delivering care in the year 2020 will be those that have invested heavily in quality care improvement today.

REFERENCES

Arndt, M., & Bigelow, B. (1998). Reengineering: Déjà vu all over again. *Health Care Management Review, 23*(3), 58–66.

Azevedo, D. (1996, August 26). Will the states get tough with HMOs? *Medical Economics,* 172–185.

Bates, D. W., Spell, N. S., Cullen, D. J., Burdick, E., Larid, N., Peterson, L. A., Small, S. D., Sweitzer, B. J., & Leape, L. L. (1997, January). The costs of adverse drug events in hospitalized patients. *Journal of the American Medical Association, 277*(4), 307–311.

Bowers, M.R., Swan, J. E., & Koehler, W. F. (1994). What attributes determine quality and satisfaction with health care delivery? *Health Care Management Review, 19*(4), 49–55.

Burns, L. R., & Beach, L. R. (1994). The quality improvement strategy. *Health Care Management Review, 19*(2), 21–31.

Chesanow, N. (1997, August 11). Making doctors' lives easier—and patients happier. *Medical Economics,* 118–131.

Dixon, R., & Trenchard, P. M. (1996). The role of precision and quality in clinical costings. *Health Care Management Review, 21*(2), 1–15.

Eddy, D. M. (1997, May/June). Balancing cost and quality in fee-for-service versus managed care. *Health Affairs, 16*(3), 162–173.

Entman, S. S., Glass, C. A., Hickson, G. B., Githens, P. B., Whetten-Goldstein, K., & Sloan, F. A. (1994). The relationship between malpractice claims history and subsequent obstetric care. *Journal of the American Medical Association, 272,* 1588–1591.

Gustafson, D. H., & Hundt, A. S. (1995, Spring). Findings of innovation research applied to quality management principles for health care. *Health Care Management Review, 20*(2), 16–33.

Hammer, M., & Champy, J. (1993). *Reengineering the corporation.* New York: Harper Business.

Heskett, J. L., Sasser, E., & Schlesinger, L. A. (1997). *The service profit chain.* New York: Free Press.

Hickson, G. B., Clayton, E. W., Githens, P. B., Sloan, F.A. (1992, March 11). Factors that prompted families to file medical malpractice claims following perinatal injuries. *JAMA. 267*(10): 1359–63.

Hickson, G. B., Clayton, E. W., Entman, S. S., Miller, C. S., Githens, P. B., Whetten-Goldstein, K., & Sloan, F. A. (1994, November 23). Obstetricians' prior malpractice experience and patients' satisfaction with care. *Journal of the American Medical Association, 272,* 1583–1587.

Ho, S. J., Chan, L., & Kidwell, R. E. (1999, Spring). The implementation of business process reengineering in American and Canadian hospitals. *Health Care Management Review, 24*(2), 19–31.

Huntington, S. (1998, February). Understanding managed care organizations' liability exposure. *Healthcare Financial Management,* 41–42.

Ingram, B. L., & Chung, R. S. (1997, Summer). Client satisfaction data and quality improvement planning in managed health care organizations. *Health Care Management Review, 22*(3), 40–52.

Joint Commission on Accreditation of Healthcare Organizations. (1996). *Accreditation manual for hospitals, volume II.* Oakbrook Terrace, IL: JCAHO.

Jun, M., Peterson, R. T., & Zsidisin, G. A. (1998, Fall). The identification and measurement of quality dimensions in health care. *Health Care Management Review, 23*(4), 81–96.

Kuttner, R. (1998, May 21). Must good HMOs go bad? Part II. *New England Journal of Medicine, 338*(22), 1625–1639.

Landon, B. E., Wilson, I. B., & Cleary, P. D. (1998, May 6). A conceptual model of the effects of health care organizations on the quality of medical care. *New England Journal of Medicine, 279*(17), 1377–1382.

LaPuma, J. (1998, March/April). Integrity in managed care: A short guide. *MGM Journal,* 53–59.

Leape, L. L. (1994, December 21). Error in medicine. *Journal of the American Medical Association, 272*(230), 1851–1857.

Leape, L .L., Lawthers, A. G., Brennan, T. A., & Johnson, W. G. (1993). Preventing medical injury. *Quality Review Bulletin, 19,* 144–149.

Lesar, T .S., Briceland, L., & Stein, D. S. (1997, January 22). Factors related to errors in medication prescribing. *Journal of the American Medical Association, 277*(4), 312–317.

Mack, J. L., File, K. M., Horwitz, J. E., & Prince, R. A. (1995). The effect of urgency on patient satisfaction. *Health Care Management Review, 20*(2), 7–15.

Manian, F. A. (1998, April 19). Should we accept mediocrity? *New England Journal of Medicine, 338*(15), 1067–1069.

Murray, D. (1996, May 28). Electronic records solved this practice's problems. *Medical Economics,* 135–147.

Orlando, M.L. (1998). Outcomes: Essential information for clinical division support: An interview with Ellen. B. White. *Journal of Healthcare Finance, 24*(3), 71–81.

Parasuraman, A., Zeithaml, V. A., & Berry, L. L. (1985, Fall). A conceptual model of service quality and its implications for future research. *Journal of Marketing, 49*(4), 41–50.

Pizzo, L. J. (1995, February 13). Ten ways to show health plans how good you are. *Medical Economics,* 48–49.

Sloan, F. A., Mergenhagen, P. M., Burfield, W. B., Bovbjerg, R. R., & Hassen, M. (1989). Medical malpractice experience of physicians: Predictable of haphazard? *Journal of the American Medical Association, 262,* 3291–3297.

Smith, H. L., Yourstone, S. A., Lorber, D., & Mann, B. (2001). Managed care and medical practice guidelines: The thorny problem of attaining physician compliance. *Advances in Health Care Management, 2,* 93–130.

Spragins, E. E. (1999, March 1). What are they hiding? *Newsweek,* 74.

Steel, K., Gertman, P. M., Crescenzi, C., & Anderson, J. (1981, March 12). Iatrogenic illness on a general medical service at a university hospital. *New England Journal of Medicine, 304*(11), 638–642.

Taylor, S. A. (1994). Distinguishing service quality from patient satisfaction in developing health care marketing strategies. *Hospital & Health Services Administration Quarterly, 39,* 221–236.

Taylor, S. L., & Capella, L. M. (1996). Hospital outshopping: Determinant attributes and hospital choice. *Health Care Management Review, 21*(4), 33–44.

Waress, B. J., Pasternak, D. P., & Smith, H. L. (1994). Determining costs associated with quality in health care delivery. *Health Care Management Review, 19*(3), 52–63.

Weil, T. P., & Battistella, R. M. (1998). A blended strategy using competitive and regulatory models. *Health Care Management Review, 23*(1), 37–45.

Woodside, A. G., Lisa, L. F., & Daly, R. T. (1989). Linking service quality, customer satisfaction and behavioral intention. *Journal of Health Care Marketing, 9*(4), 5–17.

Yasin, M. M., Czuchry, A. J., Jennings, D. L., & York, C. (1999). Managing the quality efforts in a health care setting. *Health Care Management Review, 24*(1), 45–56.

Chapter 7

Enlightened Organizations and Visionary Management

Executive Summary

Organizational and leadership skills are undeniably essential in achieving a high-performing medical group. Four focal organizational issues must be addressed:

1. Developing inspiring visions;
2. Cultivating distinctive competencies and capabilities;
3. Introducing brilliant organizational advancements; and
4. Instilling high-level incentives.

Effective leadership for exemplary medical groups will conscientiously strive to implement innovative efforts in these four areas.

Delivering the right care at the right time with kindness and quality at the lowest cost represents an overarching vision that can guide formation of fundamental strategic and tactical medical group visions. An organizational vision is essentially a preferred future or ideal that a medical group is seeking to achieve. It represents a realistic stretch of aspirations and the future embodiment of the group. The overarching vision sets a platform upon which medical group leaders define a preferred future—one that is inspirational, a basis for decision making and an aid in keeping things focused.

Cultivating distinctive competencies and capabilities implies rigorous attention to three key areas of performance:

1. Selecting the right personnel;
2. Organizing effective care delivery; and
3. Building core competencies.

High-performing organizations spend extensive time in selecting the best staff members who fit with their unique culture. Staff is then organized in a way that promotes strategy execution—the structure of a medical group should follow the guiding strategies designed to achieve the group's vision. At the center of this effort is the recognition that specific skills, talents and resources are focused on building core competencies that can become competitive advantages.

High-performing medical groups will introduce brilliant organizational advancements—startling revision in strategy or the execution of strategy that sets groups apart from other competitors. Most normal organizations tend to incrementally implement changes in strategy in response to external pressures. Medical groups do not have the luxury of plodding along with small successive changes in how they deliver services if they want to become a benchmark performer.

Finally, the high-performing medical group will seek to instill high-level incentives. Monetary incentives have always been useful in motivating behavior. However, benchmark organizations are able to derive commitment from staff not only by creatively managing those incentives but also by capitalizing on non-monetary incentives. This chapter shows how paradigm shifts can create impressive individual and organizational performance.

THE NEED FOR VISIONARY MANAGEMENT

Successful solutions to the very complex problems before the health care system require a balanced mix of familiarity with the existing system and courage to innovate without being excessively tied to present constraints. The health care dilemma in the United States will never be effectively resolved as long as we continue to bandage the widespread and increasing number of dysfunctional elements comprising the delivery setting. However, at the same time, solutions that initiate medical reform will confront significant resistance from patients and providers. Consequently, a promising approach must demonstrate courageous innovation. It should build constructively on the past and present while reengineering the future. The challenge is to understand the important components of the health system and their dysfunctional nature while remaining open to creative ideas about how these pieces might be reassembled or restructured to function more effectively (Weil, 1995).

Throughout this book we have argued that the causal factors for health care malfunctions have created a system that is no longer tolerable or affordable. The present health system has excessive costs that business, the public and consumers do not want to accept any longer, and the costs continue to outstrip inflation. The malfunctions have combined to limit access. Although those with insurance are able to receive services, there remain problems with fragmentation and coordination of services. However, there is a reality for people who lack coverage because they cannot afford health insurance, yet they earn too much to qualify for public support. The cost situation is exacerbated by service duplication. Past reimbursement has provided limited incentive for health care organizations to develop strategic alliances that encourage technology sharing. Medical technology and specialty care have also become competitive weapons that lead to further duplication. These factors have resulted in an uncomfortable mix of competing forces—solutions for one or more factors often conflict with solutions for other factors. Thus, in order to develop effective solutions that require precision fit and integration, it is necessary to look beyond simple bandages or piecemeal attempts. Fresh thinking that shifts the paradigm of health care delivery is essential if innovative solutions are to be developed with lasting value.

The vision for cutting-edge medical groups seems simple enough: Deliver the right care at the right time with kindness,

quality and low cost. All that medical groups and their physicians have to do is implement the concept. This should be the easy part, but for whatever reasons, implementation of great ideas never comes easily. The belief that health care cost-control policies can be implemented easily has been one of the government's largest stumbling blocks. Even though health policy may be crafted in such a brilliant fashion that it appears to be a certain success, glitches inevitably occur. Long after the policymakers are figuring out how to best implement the concepts, clever health care providers have determined how to beat the system. Those entrepreneurs whose ethics are on the marginal side will have devised ingenious tactics to capitalize on the policy's inherent flaws—incentives to scam the system.

When ethical health care providers respond to new policies, the range of their adaptations is considerable (Robinson, 1996). In large part, the diverse responses are due to the resources at the disposal of health care providers. Not everyone is playing on a level field. Thus, if a new policy restricts reimbursement for capital expenses, the responses by any single provider may be quite different from those of the institution down the block. Perhaps a medical group has just built a new facility with the expectation that capital costs will be covered by various reimbursements. If the policy restricts capital reimbursement, this medical group is in for trouble. Yet, if its competitor down the street has few, if any, capital costs for its facility, the competitor is in a much more favorable position.

This example only begins to touch the surface of the dilemma facing every medical group. Somehow they must respond to health care policies that constrain their activities and revenues while simultaneously achieving important organizational goals such as profitability, quality of care and asset growth. Many groups have begun a journey toward vertical integration (Shortell et al., 1994) while others have contemplated outsourcing management as a strategy to address prevailing health policies (Hill & Mullen, 1996). In effect, medical groups must manage their resources and effectively organize service delivery to enhance their ability to achieve critical goals. All of this must be completed while responding to the policies developed by third-party payors and governmental regulators. Needless to say, not every group is able to manage these chores in a way that leads to distinctive performance.

Organizational and leadership activities represent a medical group's effort to orchestrate its resources in an effort to achieve pertinent group goals and to respond to the constraints of the marketplace and to the regulators. Many physicians despise both—managers and regulators (that is, bureaucrats). Physicians often perceive that their own managers are somehow out to impede the delivery of care; their perceptions of policymakers are usually equally critical. Consequently, physicians have expressed considerable interest in management services organizations that at least superficially appear to de-emphasize management influences (Kertesz, 1998). In spite of these condemnations, high-performing medical groups can attain their goals if they utilize organizational and leadership skills/resources to their distinct benefit.

FOCAL ORGANIZATION OF ISSUES

In our view, organization and leadership make the difference between a policy implemented effectively versus a policy abused. We see organizational and leadership skills/resources within medical groups as one of the key pillars essential for achieving a reinvigorated delivery system. In fact, we do not believe that medical groups can rise to greatness unless they have cultivated and nurtured exceptional organizational talents. Experience has shown that resources do not just somehow transform themselves into something distinctive overnight. It takes brilliant strategy and careful implementation for the desired results to be achieved. Certainly, luck can play a role, but medical groups do not have the luxury of time to wait around for their luck to change and thereby suddenly enable them to achieve great results.

Figure 7.1 presents an overview of the focal organizational issues that must be effectively addressed by high-performing medical groups. First, **high-performing medical groups are able to develop inspiring visions.** As part of their strategic planning process, they formulate a view of the future—an image of the group several years down the road—that excites staff members and encourages them to deliver more than they would otherwise (Derrick & Scott, 1995). The vision instills passion in all that physicians, nurses, ancillary staff and managers do in the course of completing their jobs. The vision becomes a source of inspiration to get people through hard times, to enable them to deliver super-human effort and to keep them focused on their view of the possible.

Second, **high-performing medical groups cultivate distinctive competencies and capabilities.** The best groups do not just fill vacant positions regardless of professional level. They search for the absolute best person to fill the position(s). They seek the individual with the

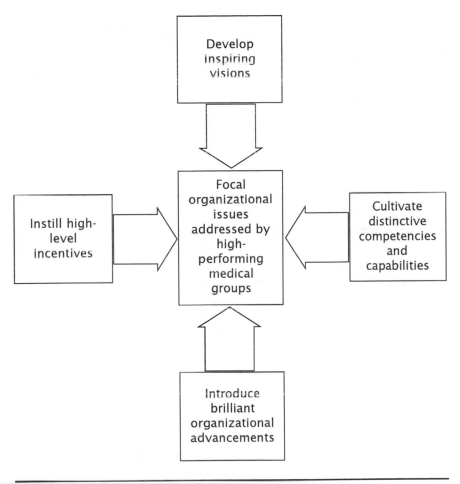

FIGURE 7.1   Focal Organization and Management Issues
in Transcendent Medical Groups

best skills, experience and education/training. They do not stop there because they also strive to retain individuals who share the same values and passion for the medical group's vision. This commitment to persevere in hiring the best staff is but one example of the extra effort put forth by high-performing medical groups to cultivate distinctive capabilities. This same tactic is repeated throughout the group's service delivery efforts as it attempts to build the finest ensemble of assets.

Third, high-performing medical groups display the ability to introduce brilliant organizational advancements. They do not follow the leader. They do not borrow tried-and-true concepts from others. They occupy the cutting edge and create models for other groups to follow. They are the first to consider a shift to for-profit status (Herbert, 1997) or to develop an integrated delivery system (Unland, 1995). The high-performing medical group is able to innovate because its entire staff is looking for opportunities to improve the service delivery process. Furthermore, people are reinforced when they enable the group to progress to an advanced level. Thus, the management of high-performing medical groups in part relies on organizational innovation and creativity.

Finally, Figure 7.1 indicates that high-performing medical groups are able to put in place higher-level incentives that encourage innovation and paradigm shifts. Through proper management of rewards and incentives, the high-performing medical group experiences a natural commitment by staff to initiate change and to improve operations. Rather than being consumed about how to sell ideas to staff—how to cajole staff into accepting a pending change—leaders of high-performing medical groups can devote their energies to positive actions critical in achieving the distinctive vision. Incentive management becomes an effective strategy for medical group improvement.

The purpose of this chapter is to emphasize that focal organizational and leadership issues must be addressed by high-performing medical groups. Many clinicians will scoff at such an idea. They only see the dysfunctional side of management. They have seen mediocre managers make care delivery a chore rather than a blessing. They have found more excuses than answers when managers have responded to their questions about impediments to care. The most brilliant idea remains only an idea until it is operationalized. The same holds true for the high performing medical groups—it is just an idea unless medical groups are able to develop inspiring visions, cultivate distinctive competencies and capabilities, introduce organizational advancement, and instill higher-level incentives.

Vision as Beacon for the High-Performing Group

The right care at the right time with kindness and quality at the lowest cost represents a landmark vision that high-performing medical groups will focus on in their efforts to become leaders in the field. In many respects, this vision represents a beacon for the health care field and an inspiration for providers as they contemplate exactly what sort of mark—what kind of indelible legacy—they intend to leave behind when their time in the profession is over. Some may think that this contemplation of the future is wasted philosophizing—that medical groups really need to address current problems rather than some unattainable, distant objective. Given the particularly nasty problems that besiege the health care field, these apologists must be granted some credence. However, it is sad to think that the centuries of human effort and personal sacrifice in medicine and health must be handed over to those who see only limitations, roadblocks and obstacles rather than the bright promise of distinctive health care.

As long as there are physicians, nurses, ancillary staff, administrators, patients and other concerned individuals in health care who truly believe they can make substantive improvements in health delivery and people's lives, then the vision of a high-performing group retains legitimacy. It serves as a guiding beacon for those medical groups that are not ready to capitulate but that are committed to fighting the good fight. Additionally, the inspiring vision serves as a foundation for medical groups as they consider the paths and options before them. In effect, the inspiring vision serves as a boilerplate from which each medical group can establish its distinctive aspirations and identity.

INSPIRING MEDICAL GROUP VISIONS

An inspiring vision is the primary beacon for medical groups, but it must be accompanied by a specific vision of how each organization intends to be distinctive—unique—for its service area and set of resources (Bart & Tabone, 1999). This suggests that medical groups should develop organizational visions that serve to inspire patients, personnel and communities. Figure 7.2 conveys the important attributes of effective visions and how these organizational visions serve as a functional source of inspiration.

For many medical groups, the idea of pursuing the right care at the right time with kindness, quality and low cost should be sufficient as a set of guidelines for decision making and inspiration. However, such a lofty goal may be too conceptual in the course of organizing services and managing the implementation of care delivery to achieve the goal. Thus, for some groups it is appropriate to take a step down in conceptualization by focusing on an organizational vision that is more

What Is an Organizational Vision?

- A preferred future or ideal to achieve;
- A concept of the desirable achieved by capitalizing on opportunities;
- A realistic stretch of aspirations; and
- The future embodiment of an organization.

A vision achieves its inspiration from

Attributes that Make Visions Important

- They inspire people by providing a picture of lofty objectives.
- They serve as a rallying point, glue or common bond.
- They convey a vivid image of a preferred future, thereby facilitating decisions.
- They provide a basis for aligning people with diverse values, views and perspectives.
- They communicate the imagination and convictions of the collective body.

Attributes of Effective Visions

- They are challenging.
- They are long-term oriented but decidedly achievable.
- They are inspirational.
- They provide an anchor and basis for decision making.
- They keep things focused.

FIGURE 7.2   The Inspiration of Organizational Visions

specific to (or concrete for) short-term operations. Typically, an organizational omission defines the organizational mission, which defines the organizational purpose or reason for being in the short-run or present. Both the vision and mission provide direction, as suggested in Sidebar 7.1. As medical groups begin discussions on what their unique

SIDEBAR 7.1

The Rationale for Hospital Mission Statements

Bart and Tabone (1998) studied 103 Canadian hospitals and their mission statements to ascertain the extent to which the mission statements are aligned with the rationale that led to the development of the mission statement in the first place. With a survey questionnaire that generated a response rate of 20.8 percent, the hospital respondents employ, on average, 1,010 staff members and generates an average revenue of $53 million. The average surplus generated from options is $115,000 on an asset base worth $44 million, on average. The findings from this study indicate that managers of the not-for-profit hospitals express a prevailing consensus on what the primary rationales for their hospital missions should be:

- To provide a common direction or purpose;
- To promote shared values;
- To define the scope of business;
- To motivate and inspire employees;
- To create behavior standards;
- To enable employees to identify with the organization;
- To address the needs of external stakeholders;
- To provide a basis for allocating resources;
- To refocus an organization in crisis; and
- To enable the CEO to assert control.

The top three rationales—to provide common direction, to promote shared values and to define the scope of business—were the dominant mission drivers. It is interesting to observe that much less emphasis was expressed by the managers regarding the mission as a framework for resource allocation. It is possible that they view the strategic objectives and strategies of their strategic plan as the main framework for decisions regarding resources.

Bart and Tabone argue that, at least in Canadian not-for-profit hospitals, managers may not be using the best rationales when developing their mission statements. The implications are that a faulty mission statement may therefore be created—a statement that does not accurately guide

continued

organizational efforts or that correctly focuses organizational resources in the most effective manner. They recommend that more attention should be directed to aligning mission statement with mission rationale.

Source: Adapted from C. K. Bart & J. C. Tabone. (1998). Mission statement rationales and organizational alignment in the not-for-profit health care sector. *Health Care Management Review, 23*(4), 54–69.

vision may embody, the guidelines shown in Figure 7.2 should be quite fruitful in defining a challenging, yet achievable vision.

The first significant point for vision setting in Figure 7.2 relates to the general definition or conceptualization of what an organizational vision incorporates (Bart & Tabone, 1999). Typically, an organizational vision is a preferred future or an ideal to achieve. For example, a medical group may define its vision as, "the preferred medical clinic of choice in the state," or "the most accessible specialty provider for managed care." These statements communicate the intentions of the medical group to achieve something beyond the ordinary in their service delivery. The intention is to attain this ideal at some future point in time.

An organizational vision can also be considered a concept of the desirable that is reached by capitalizing on opportunities. The medical group defines what it perceives as desirable as well as stipulating which opportunities it will take advantage of to arrive at that goal. For example, assume a group has decided that it wants to provide state-of-the-art cardiology care at low cost with highest satisfaction to the maximum number of patients. Having identified the concept of the desirable, the vision acts as a framework for choosing among opportunities to contract with managed care plans for cardiology services. Managed care plans A (40,000 lives), B (150,000 lives) and C (85,000 lives) request a proposal for services from the group. How does the group's vision help it to prepare proposals for these managed care plans?

Superficially, it could be argued that the group should invest most effort in preparing the proposal for plan B because it covers the most lives. However, the vision provides much more guidance than that upon closer examination. What is the age composition of each plan? What is the cardiology service utilization experience of each plan? How does the group's strategies for achieving low cost mesh with the strategies and tactics employed by the plans? These are only a few of the pertinent questions suggested by the vision for the group's effort in preparing contract proposals.

The vision takes the issue of proposal development even further than suggested by the preceding questions. If the medical group in question really wants to reach the maximum number of lives, it must give serious consideration to responding competitively to all opportunities. Is there any reason to not prepare a response to any of the requests? Is there synergy that might unfold if two or more plans are successfully attained? Is there inordinate risk to the other aspirations and goals of the medical group? These are legitimate questions that can be answered due to the guidelines set forth in the vision statement.

Figure 7.2 indicates that an organizational vision represents a realistic stretch of aspirations. In this respect, a vision defines a challenging, yet reachable goal. Such a stretch should be attainable in a three-to-five-year time frame; that is, the organization will have some difficulty in reaching that goal if it does not make a significant effort over a several-year period. At the same time, the goal or final state should relate directly to strategic objectives that have been defined for the intervening years. Thus, the goal of doubling revenues to $10 million within five years is not consistent with a strategic objective of increasing revenues 10 percent every year. A compounded 10 percent increase of revenues on a $5 million base is only $8 million.

Medical groups must not only set a realistic stretch of aspirations, but they must do so in a fashion that is consistent with the more lofty inspirational target. Therefore, a medical group that sets its target as being recognized as the leading medical provider in a major metropolitan area has not quite captured the essence of what it means to be a high-performing group. **The vision for high-performing groups is not only to be recognized as a leader among caregivers, but also to be recognized for shaping the health care delivery system in fundamentally new ways—dramatically lower cost, startling provider productivity, exceptional patient satisfaction through a unique covenant, cutting-edge accessibility, or seamless connections with providers who might otherwise be viewed as competitors.**

Finally, Figure 7.2 indicates that a high-performing medical group uses a vision as a figurative portrayal of the organization—the future embodiment of the medical group. The vision attempts to paint a profile of what the organization will resemble after a certain period of time down the road. It is a snapshot of what the group will look like when it has undergone the transformation process—when it has transcended beyond the commonplace to a position of leadership. This visual representation is concrete enough for all constituents—particularly staff—to understand the primary goals to which they are working. However, it is nonspecific enough that it has a mystique and sufficient latitude for clarification as the group achieves intermediate steps or goals along the way.

The precise composition of a vision statement varies enormously. In a study of vision statements from medium-sized corporations, Larwood, Falbe, Kriger and Miesing (1995) discovered a wide range of statements in terms of their composition and content. Examples included:

- Be a major force in high-performance banking in the community bank arena;
- Be the recognized world leader in national security space system architecture and engineering;
- Double in size within five years;
- Be the leading African-American-owned promotional and public relations firm in the United States;
- Create an environment in which satisfied customers, quality products and bottom-line profits go hand-in-hand; and
- Be a survivor and prosper in a heavily and unfairly regulated industry.

As these statements suggest, there is little agreement in practice about what a vision statement might incorporate.

Health care organizations, particularly medical groups, may use the preceding examples to their advantage when crafting a vision statement. Promising vision statement options for medical groups include the following:

- Be the preferred medical group for nephrology care in the state;
- Be the largest managed care provider that offers the best care at the lowest price with the most satisfied customers;
- Create a medical group that is recognized as having the leading experts in orthopedic medicine;

- Become the medical group of choice for family medicine; and

- Double the number of patients we serve within five years without adversely affecting the quality of care.

As these examples for medical groups demonstrate, there is substantial flexibility for crafting a vision statement that captures the unique qualities of the group while also establishing an inspirational target to achieve.

Attributes That Make Visions Important

Having defined what constitutes an organizational vision, it is equally relevant to review the attributes that give visions their significance. Figure 7.2 indicates that visions achieve their inspirational qualities from certain attributes. Several factors come into play as far as how a vision attains importance.

First, visions inspire people by providing a picture of lofty objectives. In the course of providing services on a daily basis, it is all too easy for monotony to creep into even the most motivated professional, care provider or medical group. Routine may bring with it a sense of alienation from personal objectives and the awareness of contribution to valuable medical efforts. A vision can often help people refocus their attention and motivation. The vision depicts a lofty set of objectives or a goal that the medical group is striving to attain. Progress will occur in incremental steps rather than by leaps and bounds—such is the nature of most service delivery efforts. Whenever staff displays a sense of wandering or lack of focus, it is the inspirational vision that can redirect its ambitions, attention and commitment.

Because visions provide a picture of desired results that a medical group wishes to achieve, they also serve as a rallying point, glue or common bond as staff members share their belief in a concerted or team effort. Visions help to bring people together—even people who may have had rather intense differences of opinion about medical care issues. By encouraging medical group personnel to remember the shared vision, managers are able to constructively direct attention toward positive aspirations. This emphasis on a positive goal defuses tensions and clarifies the reason for delivering care in the first place. In this respect, medical group visions are extremely valuable because they focus motivation toward a common hurdle or challenge that may not be overcome without a concerted effort.

A third important aspect of visions is their ability to convey a vivid image of a preferred future, thereby facilitating decisions. Simply put, it is tremendously easier to make decisions when you possess a concept of which direction a medical group should be heading. The vision provides the framework for decisions. Can the same be said for a medical group's mission? The answer to this question is yes. However, there is an important difference in the image communicated by mission and vision statements. The vision attempts to convey a particularly inspirational goal while the mission actually depicts the existing aspirations of the group. Timing makes a difference—present versus future—as well as the emotional constant—inspirational versus descriptive. In the end, both the mission and the vision facilitate decisions. However, it is the vision portraying such a vivid image of the future that has practicality in the near term.

A vision is also important because it provides a basis for aligning people with diverse values, views and perspectives. This does not necessarily imply that a vision can reduce the degree of disagreement between two (or more) sharply held concepts of the desirable. On the contrary, a distinctive vision is often a contributor to individuals recognizing their differences rather than reducing their differences. Instead, a vision has special merit because it helps define the values that a medical group represents; the views and interpretations of issues that the staff is prone to possess; and the interpretations of issues relevant to medical care delivery. This ability to clarify what the group values is particularly important in ensuring that professionals with similar values, views and perspectives remain with and are attracted to the group.

There is a downside to the cultivation of a dominant mindset. The phenomenon of group thinking may make a medical group vulnerable to important environmental changes that go unrecognized because of the prevailing thinking patterns, processes and conclusions. There are, however, many conventions that can be employed to reduce the potential dysfunctional presence of group thinking (for example, the use of outside experts/consultants, issue debates wherein two opposing views are aired before decisions are made, and so forth). Without an organization-wide effort to create a fundamental value system, a medical group can have significant trouble in resolving difficult issues. From our experience, it is more difficult to nurture a common value system than it is to obtain divergent opinions. Furthermore, exemplary organizations have demonstrated the capacity to establish and capitalize on a dominant value system (for example, IBM, McDonalds, Intel), whereas organizations with highly divergent values internally tend to achieve more modest results. In sum, an organization culture with a dominant value system is usually one that reconciles conflict, nurtures innovation, motivates staff and produces respected return on investment.

A final attribute that lends importance to medical group visions is their ability to communicate the imagination and convictions of the collective staff. **A vision is often as much a reason why a physician should not join a group as it is a reason why she or he should leave.** In this sense, the vision helps potential medical staff members and other personnel from joining the wrong organization. Each person who is employed by a medical group uses precious energy and effort from others as he or she tries to establish a fit within the group. A vision statement can reduce the number of false starts and, hence, conserve energy, emotion and effort as far as integrating providers within the organizational team. In the same line of thinking, an organizational vision can help those who are already involved with the group to rethink their fit with the prevailing culture. It can provide a convenient soundingboard and conversation initiative to encourage those who do not fit within the group to reconsider other external opportunities.

Attributes of Effective Visions

Figure 7.2 suggests that visions achieve their inspirational qualities from a number of attributes. Medical groups that are able to incorporate these attributes within their visions and vision statements are better positioned as far as effectively applying visionary guidance in operating and strategic venues. As Figure 7.2 indicates, effective visions are challenging. They encourage medical groups to reach beyond their status quo toward a more accomplished future. For example, a medical group may have added two pediatricians in the last year in rounding out its strategic thrust to become the preferred provider of pediatric services in a major metropolitan city. In the midst of self-congratulation, the senior pediatrician asks what the group will strive to achieve next. Without a challenging vision this question will go unanswered. Ideally, the group would have rearticulated its vision, perhaps to set a challenging goal of being the preferred provider of pediatric services in the state.

Another attribute of effective visions is their recognition of the present and linkage to the future. Effective visions are long-term oriented, but they are decidedly achievable. Thus, the medical group that constructs an image of its future as the preferred provider of pediatric services in the state explicitly incorporates the present with the future; that is, the group has sufficient resources and momentum to actually achieve the preferred goal of being the state's preferred pediatric services provider in the future. It may take several years to unfold the specific strategies that enable the medical group to attain this vision, but nonetheless, the goal is reachable.

Effective visions are also notable for their inspirational qualities. The pediatric group that has grown slowly in patient load and physician capability over a 10-year period may well reflect that it will never become anything other than an also-ran competitor. **The purpose of the vision is to ignite excitement, enthusiasm and confidence in building a better medical group.** If the physicians in a group do not set their sights high, then they will never reach the point of distinction. If agreement can be reached on an inspiring future, the vision can motivate staff to expend tremendous effort, ingenuity and skill in reaching for a future target where the medical group becomes an institutional legend.

While visions play an important role in motivating people to excel, they also have a very practical side that assists the group's operations. Effective visions provide an anchor and basis for decision making. The vision helps communicate what the group is all about and therefore tends to keep people on track. For example, if a pediatric group is striving to become the state's preferred provider for pediatric services, this anchor helps the group assess the opportunity to affiliate with a multispecialty group practice. Unless the affiliation agreement contributes to the fundamental vision, the pediatric group must assess the opportunity as one that should be passed by in the course of strategic options.

Finally, Figure 7.2 indicates that effective visions help to keep things focused. There are many distractions in the daily delivery of medical services. Effective visions help physicians, nurses, ancillary staff and managers keep their eyes on the prize—the preferred future that they covet. For example, a physician in a pediatric group may attend a wonderful continuing medical education session at a professional meeting. She returns confident that the concept of patient care contracts is perfect for resolving many of the problems the group has encountered with patients' parents regarding aftercare. Her colleagues are attuned to the trends in medical education, especially the tendency for professional conferences to peddle the latest medical and management fads. However, in this instance, the vision for the group helps the physician convince her colleagues that a patient care contract is consistent with better medical care. The vision keeps the assessment (of the patient care contract) focused on providing the right care at the right time with kindness, quality and low cost.

CULTIVATING DISTINCTIVE COMPETENCIES AND CAPABILITIES

In order for organizational and managerial practices within medical groups to successfully facilitate care, there must be a corresponding effort to cultivate distinctive competencies and capabilities. Mediocre talent produces mediocre results. While this level of performance was tolerated and even encouraged within the health care system of past decades, all signs point to a revolution in thinking and in constraints. Medical groups that expect to maintain their complacency about how their operations are organized and managed are in for a big surprise. The evolving health care environment will demand razor-sharp operations by all providers. The also-rans and those who were content to produce less-than-impressive results will vanish. This applies to both individual practitioners and to organizations.

Figure 7.3 illustrates three critical managerial issues essential in nurturing the high-performing medical group. All three issues are related to cultivating distinctive competencies and capabilities. Medical groups will argue that they have always sought to select the right personnel, to build core competencies and to organize effectively in their service delivery. However, the health care environment that is beginning to surface suggests that these efforts must be substantially upgraded and intensified for the challenges to come. Thus, medical groups must revisit what it means to build distinctive competencies and capabilities.

First, the high-performing medical group will require the right personnel who work together (Mintzberg, 1997). In the past, the right personnel were often viewed through the lens of who was best trained in their profession and who might fit best personality-wise into the group's culture. These qualities will still retain importance in the years to come. However, medical groups will use several very

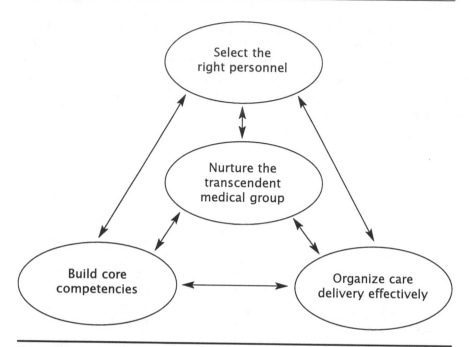

FIGURE 7.3 Cultivating Distinctive Competencies and Capabilities

different lenses as they determine which potential staff members they want to employ. The coming health care context requires more than people who fit professionally and are compatible personality-wise. Medical groups in the present and future will need individuals who are able to work on multidisciplinary teams, who demonstrate they are committed to improving services constantly, who respond to group incentives, who think of customers/patients first, and who are adaptable in changing with the new strategies that medical groups must introduce.

The profile that emerges on personnel is a decidedly different one from that currently used when selecting staff to join a medical group. Consequently, the implication is that medical groups will have to spend more time and effort in determining the best candidate within the available pool. The implication is that physicians, nurses and ancillary support staff will all be involved in interviewing and assessing candidates. This may seem heretical to some physicians, that nonphysicians would evaluate physicians' potential for a medical group. However, if multidisciplinary teams are to be conceived and implemented, compatible team members are essential. Aspiring candidates will discover that they must present a more comprehensive set of information about their skills, capabilities, attitudes, experiences and results. The end result will be more careful attention to selecting the right personnel—those people who will enable the group to deliver the desired results.

High-performing medical groups will face the challenge of organizing care more effectively (Kralewski, et al., 1998). To many physicians and other clinicians, this emphasis on organization may seem tangential to the real task of delivering care. Does all that management and organization talk just obscure and hinder the real action in attending to patients? While that sort of perception may have been true in the past, providers will discover that there is substantial value in organizing effectively to deliver services. In fact, they will realize that without advanced organizational and managerial practices, medical care delivery will be less efficient and effective. If care costs more due to inefficiencies or due to poor quality, a medical group and its staff will find that the future is very tenuous. Consequently, clinicians will develop a new appreciation for and embrace effective organization and management principles.

Medical groups will find that to organize effectively means relinquishing the traditional structures that have come to characterize health care organizations (Burns, 1996). The prime issue in organizing is not who is most important and around whom the organization is structured; but rather, how do we best organize to serve clients/patients/customers? A prevalent rule that has surfaced in the strategy literature is structure should follow strategy. Thus, medical groups will determine a strategy for service delivery that effectively guides how they organize.

Finally, Figure 7.3 indicates that the high-performing medical group will be nurtured by building core competencies. Each group that aspires to success must develop specialized skills, talents, resources and technical expertise that help to differentiate it from other medical groups (Lowes, 1996). Not every medical group can be the preferred provider of general medical care or pediatric care or cardiology. Medical groups want to avoid having a reputation for delivering acceptable care in all areas but having no distinctive characteristics. Acceptable care will not cut it in the future of health care. Medical groups must be able to demonstrate that they are the best in an area of care.

INTRODUCING BRILLIANT ORGANIZATIONAL ADVANCES

Every health care administrator, whether hospital administrator, medical practice executive, long-term care administrator or managed care director, is responsible for ensuring that the absolute maximum benefit is obtained from the assets of his or her organization. Their job is to make certain that the resources with which they have been entrusted produce the most output and achieve the highest quality, lowest cost, highest net revenue and best customer satisfaction. This is a big responsibility. However, at the same time, these managers must also look for ways in which to improve not only the operations of their organizations, but the strategic direction as well (MGMA, 1998). Day-to-day operations tend to erode the amount of time managers may devote to critical strategic thinking and organizational renewal processes that possess far-ranging implications. Unfortunately, it is precisely these longer-run issues that have the most significant ramifications for health care organizations and their ability to prosper.

Medical group managers now understand that they can no longer be content with running a tight ship. The redefinition of medical and health care confronts each medical group daily. Sound management practices and skillful strategizing will always be needed. However, medical practice executives are now being held accountable not only for stellar operating and strategic performance, but they must demonstrate the ability to integrate and innovate throughout the care delivery process (Devers, et al., 1994). In essence, it is insufficient to just be a good manager; now the expectations have risen. Medical practice executives must also consistently display the ability to design and implement creative advances on both the operational and strategic sides of the business.

This new expectation is actually an imperative. Medical groups cannot afford to do less than continually reinvent what it means to deliver the best of care at low cost with kindness and high quality. Those groups whose managers are unable to continually inject brilliant advances in the operations and strategy underlying service delivery will eventually pay the price whether through dismal, modest performance, or eventual demise. In this respect, medical practice executives must turn up their organization and management skills several notches if they intend to succeed in the tumultuous health care arena.

Figure 7.4 depicts the shift in managerial acumen, orientation and results that are becoming imperative in the medical care field. Two comparative approaches to managing are displayed—the traditional management approach and the high-performance approach. Under the traditional approach to managing, a series of interventions, reconfigurations, redesigns or reengineering, or solutions are attempted to solve a problem. The issue, or problem, is attacked incrementally in a series of linear adjustments to the care delivery process. Over time, the group does make progress in addressing the issue at hand. The question is whether this progress is rapid enough and whether the changes are sufficient to produce the desired outcomes.

An illustration may explain this sequence best. Assume that a medical group has the best intentions of responding to rising health care costs. In its affiliation with a managed care plan, a consensus is reached that every effort will be made to avoid unnecessary surgery. If the medical group specializes in ophthalmology, a target medical condition that receives attention for cost control is cataract surgery. The managed care plan and the medical group agree to minimize unnecessary surgical procedures for cataracts. Of course, the definition of what constitutes necessary surgery is complex and open to the judgment of the group's physicians. Nonetheless, organizationally, the medical group coordinates its service delivery efforts with this target in mind. If the programmatic thrust is effectively managed, the medical group will be able to deliver the most necessary care (that is, surgery only when absolutely necessary), the managed care plan will be able to hold down its costs, patients will incur low costs (for the managed care coverage they receive) and the medical group will be able to retain its contract.

With these achievements in place, the medical group and managed care plan attempt to ratchet the process up another level. They seek to promote prevention among the patient population. Health promotion becomes a panacea for health maintenance. In concert, the medical group and managed care plan design and implement a program aimed at eye care and the prevention of eye-related diseases. Over time, the program may have an impact to the extent that the health costs for this patient population are reduced.

The traditional management approach to care delivery follows a linear sequence of progressive improvements. Many times this is the best approach because of the tendency for people to resist change. Most often an incremental solution of a series of smaller problems can

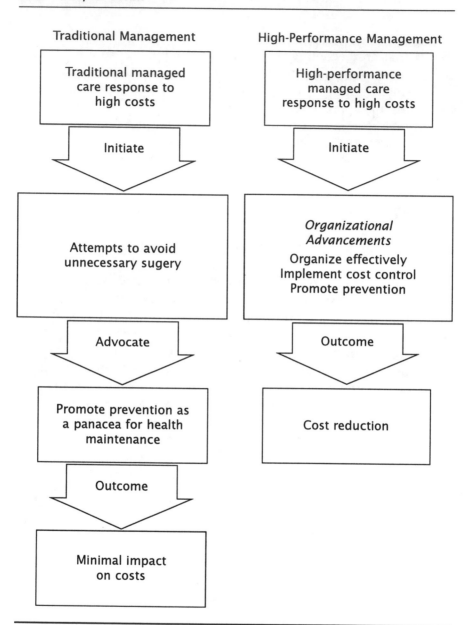

FIGURE 7.4 Comparative Advances in Managing Care

lead to large results. Will this traditional approach deliver the kind of outcomes that medical groups need today? Will successive improvements provide the sorts of return and advancement in care delivery required to address the imperatives accompanying health care reform?

Figure 7.4 suggests that another approach to managing care delivery problems is feasible. A high-performance management strategy initiates comprehensive treatment rather than sequential improvements. Returning to the medical group that has contracted with the managed care plan for eye care, a more far-ranging effort could be implemented to achieve better results in less time. The high-performing group initiates a host of organizational advancements simultaneously. The group and managed care plan cannot wait for a series of programmatic thrusts to unfold. They, and their patients, need results today.

The medical group decides it must address eye care costs in a sweeping manner within its service delivery efforts. First, the group organizes the manner in which care is provided. One (or more) physician is assigned the responsibility of completing all cataract surgeries. She is delegated authority to form a care delivery team that must produce a high number of surgeries at the lowest possible cost. The team is responsible for determining how these outcomes will be achieved; that is, how they will organize and operate in order to achieve the specified objectives.

Second, the medical group implements a comprehensive cost-control effort. By coordinating with the managed care plan, the group identifies the cost thresholds that the managed care plan desires. However, this is only one element in the group's efforts to control costs. The challenge presented by the care plan offers an opportunity for the group to rethink, redesign and achieve cost control in many areas. Third, the group also designs and puts into operation a health promotion program aimed at reducing the need for eye care services over the long run. Clearly, the promotion program will have some impact, but it cannot take the demand for eye care services to zero. The sum of these three organizational advances, introduced simultaneously, is significant cost reduction. The high-performing medical group is able to achieve a larger impact more quickly because it intensifies its management effort.

Realistically, medical groups and their managers will not always be able to introduce significant advances in service delivery with certain success. Nonetheless, the goal is to advance management beyond the ordinary. Figure 7.5 conveys this thought as the progressive introduction of brilliant organizational advances. An initial paradigm shift occurs that sets the process in motion. Perhaps it is the medical group's commitment to controlling health care costs. The paradigm shift sets in motion a series of strategies.

Strategy #1 is designed to improve operations management by identifying high-cost services; that is, the group analyzes its cost of services to identify the most costly service areas (per resource input). Strategy #2 focuses cost control in one service delivery area. As it reaches success, Strategy #3 comes into play as the tactics are operationalized throughout the highest-cost service areas and all other points in which costs can be controlled. The initial paradigm shift generates another revolution in service delivery. The subsequent paradigm shift enables the medical group to go beyond internal efforts at cost control to rethinking the sort of physicians and other providers that should be added to the staff. The group implements a new policy of hiring providers for their demonstrated record of cost-control results. This criterion is added to the list of criteria for selection; it may be favorably weighted compared to other criteria.

The progressive introduction of brilliant organizational advancements shown in Figure 7.5 does differ significantly from the traditional sequence of managerial improvements depicted in Figure 7.4 in at least two ways. First, traditional management approaches take good ideas and then applies them sequentially. In contrast, high-performing approaches begin with a paradigm shift—a revolution in the design of care delivery or the reengineering of the entire service delivery process even though the process may just focus on one procedure, medical condition or subspecialty area. Second, traditional management approaches do not generate subsequent brilliant organizational and managerial advances. Paradigm shifts are reinforcing. Their results tend to encourage further experimentation and bold change necessary to attack tough problems—the sort of problems that must be addressed if medical care is to advance.

INSTILLING HIGH-LEVEL INCENTIVES

If there is any doubt that the health care system has methodically driven health care managers and care providers to the point that there is less incentive to work hard in delivering care, then it is proper to

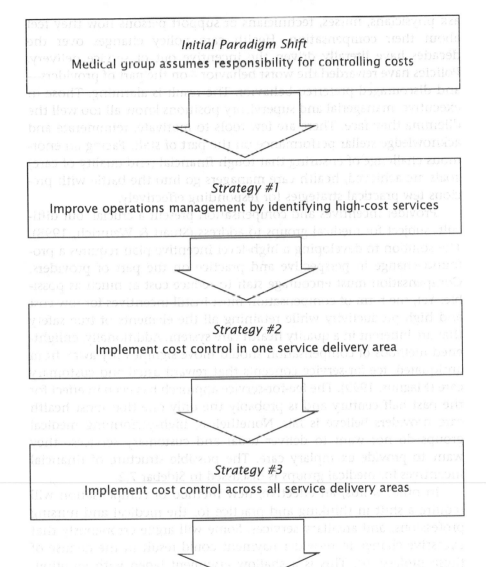

FIGURE 7.5   Progressive Introduction of Brilliant
Organizational Advancements

ask physicians, nurses, technicians or support persons how they feel about their compensation. Health care policy changes over the decades have literally driven the incentive out of service delivery. Policies have rewarded the worst behavior—on the part of providers—and discouraged preferred behavior. The result is alarming. Those in executive, managerial and supervisory positions know all too well the dilemma they face. There are few tools to motivate, remunerate and acknowledge stellar performance on the part of staff. Facing an enormous challenge of ensuring that tough financial (and quality of care) goals are achieved, health care managers go into the battle with precious few practical strategies for responding effectively.

Provider incentives and compensation present a crucial, but difficult, subject for medical groups to address (Stuart & Weinrich, 1998). The solution to developing a high-level incentive plan requires a profound change in perspective and practice on the part of providers. Compensation must encourage staff to reduce cost as much as possible. Yet, the form of compensation must instill incentives for low cost and high productivity while retaining all the elements of true safety that are inherent in a quality health care system. Additionally, enlightened methods of compensation should move significantly away from antiquated, fee-for-service concepts that reward usual and customary care (Magnus, 1999). The fee-for-service approach has been in effect for the past half century and is probably the only one that most health care providers believe is fair. Nonetheless, high-performing medical groups do not want to deliver usual and customary services—they want to provide exemplary care. The possible structure of financial incentives for medical groups is discussed in Sidebar 7.2.

In other words, an effective, new method of compensation will require a shift in thinking and practice for the medical and nursing professions, and ancillary services. Some will argue erroneously that excessive change in provider payment could result in the demise of these professions. This is a shallow argument laden with emotion. Changes are necessary because, frankly, health care costs too much. No one aware of the budget battles in the country and efforts to balance the budget in the future can be complacent about how health care will or will not be funded in the future. It is an enormous problem. The amount of money spent on health care will not increase as it has in the past and may well be reduced. If one looks on the other side at the literature on health maintenance organizations and capitation payment, the advice and arguments concern how to negotiate

SIDEBAR 7.2
Financial Incentives for Physicians in HMOs

Mangus (1999) proposed a conceptual framework for physician incentives—positive and negative—in health maintenance organizations. Several research studies have indicated that financial incentives can have a powerful effect in influencing physician practice behaviors—a more powerful impact than nonmonetary initiatives such as utilization review or preauthorization policies (Egdahl & Taft, 1986; Kwon, 1996). There is clearly a fine distinction between financial incentives that spur on desired behaviors by physicians in their practices versus undesired clinical behaviors. This ethical dilemma does not suggest that all financial incentives should be discarded, but rather that internal controls for accountability and review are appropriately created and implemented by participating HMOs.

Physicians may be exposed to two sorts of financial incentives by HMOs. First, there are base compensation plans that affect practice:

Compensation Plan	Ramifications
Salary	Favors stability of behavior and possibly a restrained use of resources but also may lower productivity and shortened working hours
Capitation	Motivates efficiency and a decreased use of resources (possibly an underuse)
Fee-for-service	Creates incentives for an increase in services and resource use (possibly an overuse)

The base compensation plan sets a foundation from which the system of financial incentives can be applied.

Magnus proposes two opposing incentives, each with two possible manifestations in the contemporary HMO environment:

Incentive Type	Rationale
Positive Incentives Bonuses	• Encourages greater effort and higher performance and productivity • Can be calculated as a predetermined, fixed-dollar amount, a fixed percentage of the HMO's surplus, a function of physicians' productivity, or a function of physicians' scores on patient satisfaction surveys

continued

Incentive Type	Rationale
Profit Sharing	• Promotes a sense of investment and ownership in the organization • May be largely symbolic in value because of the remote link between profits and an individual physician's performance
Negative Incentives Withholdings	• Creates sensitivity to the costs of specialist referrals, lab services, surgery, etc. • May be returned depending on the performance of a referral fund or the HMO as a whole • Is most likely to affect primary care physicians acting as gatekeepers
Penalties	• Conveys strong management disapproval to physicians • Magnifies the impact of withholdings • Includes decreases in capitation, increases in withholdings, reductions in distributions from fund surpluses and liens on future earnings

The goal is to create a set of balanced incentives—a goal that is very elusive in practice.

Source: Adapted from S. A. Magnus. (1999). Physicians' financial incentives in five dimensions. *Health Care Management Review, 24*(1), 45–56.

higher capitation rates, how to obtain a mix of patients that will require less care, or how to increase productivity in the medical sense (that is, having doctors see more patients). These cutting-edge ideas do not relate to the fundamental problem—reducing the cost of the care that is necessary.

Toward Higher-Level Incentives

At the present time, capitation has reduced some costs, but in ways that inadvertently harm the patient. This is not surprising because health care providers have not had experience with increasing productivity and do not know how to reduce costs. The goal is to reduce the cost of what is done, not reduce what is done. A new plan for compensating providers must be first a coherent, comprehensive system that is based on efficiency and costs less for the same results. This goal can only be achieved by increasing productivity. Health care providers must be rewarded for exactly what is desired, what is high quality, and what is efficient. Obviously, this means they must not be rewarded for doing more or less, but for performing the right care at the right time. The end point, not the process, needs to be utilized to evaluate results. Finally, compensation for a health care provider should never be affected by what is done for a single patient. Compensation should not be higher or lower (that is, negative bonus) based on whether a single patient has or does not have an operation. If necessary, the operation should be done. If unnecessary, it should not be done; but a doctor should be able to make the best clinical decision without regard as to whether he or she will be rewarded or punished financially.

Implementation of creative compensation plans will be difficult. Health care providers, doctors and hospitals tend to focus on what used to be and try to return to the past. Thinking of ways to do an operation less expensively will be a foreign exercise and uncomfortable. Moreover, because there are regulated institutions and professions, rules and boundaries based on past experience will interfere with a plan to reduce costs. Consider the following example. There are many instances in which a diagnostic test is performed by hand and evaluated by a physician with regard to normality. Now a machine can often perform the test and indicate whether it is normal or abnormal. Even if normal, the reading has to be checked by a physician. Of course, if abnormal, a medical evaluation may be necessary. If the computer indicates that the test is normal, it is expensive and inefficient for a physician to reread the test. Physician time could be better and more productively spent in other areas. However, compensation must provide incentives to physicians to redirect their time.

An experienced multidisciplinary team headed by a physician is probably the most efficient approach to achieving high productivity and low cost. Individuals on the team need to be trained exactly for what they do, and there should be maximum use of nonphysician personnel. Protocols and procedures should be developed for all functions by all members of the team. Concepts of medical manufacturing and six sigma should be utilized. All of these elements are critical for success. However, they alone are not sufficient. A system of incentives must be implemented. For example, bonuses might be distributed so that each member of the team receives the same percentage bonus. The leaders should not be the only ones rewarded. It may also be desirable in the beginning to reward each team by a fixed amount for reducing costs. It is important to emphasize again that we are talking about basic costs, not the money the employers of the team receive. To the extent the costs are reduced, there is more net gain to offset capitation. The team members might be told, for example, that if they reduce costs by a certain amount, the team will receive 40 percent of that amount the first year and 20 percent the second year. How costs are reduced needs to be open and agreed upon so that there is no reduction in clinical quality.

A group or team approach to defining incentive distribution is initially perplexing but not altogether impractical. There have been many instances in which, by utilizing team function and brainstorming, the same doctor has become five times as efficient. This means that from the doctor's compensation point of view, the cost is theoretically one-fifth of the former cost. In most operating rooms where different surgeons follow each other, it may turn out that two major operations can be completed in an operating room in half a day (for example, four per day). In one institution where two or three gynecologic surgeons perform all the operations for a gynecologic department, each is assigned one or two operating rooms. The surgeons routinely completed nine or ten major procedures in a day. This is two-fold increase in productivity. Without a large group, no gynecologist would have enough operations to make this practical; but with clinical care moving to managed care, this type of organization may become practical and desirable. In short, operative quality and cost control will improve if the best surgeon does 40 operations a week rather than 40 surgeons doing one operation per week.

Soon the focus will also be directed to determining the value of a procedure in compensation terms. What is a procedure worth? Basically, it is worth what it costs to have the procedure done effectively. If a first-year resident (after six months of specialty training) can do the procedure well, the cost in professional compensation would be calculated from a fraction (that is, time for the procedure) of his or her salary, not the usual and customary fees assigned to a private doctor. This means that if the system becomes more efficient and fewer doctors are required, physician compensation could be markedly reduced.

In conclusion, several things are evident. Due to cost problems, reimbursement for medical care will not rise as providers would otherwise hope. Certainly, provider payment will not rise in proportion to the number of new patients coming into the system. Technology and scientific discoveries will tend to increase what can be done in a positive sense and, therefore, increase costs. When considered carefully, it is evident that it is in the personal interest of every physician and provider to adapt and try to work out a new compensation system. From the point of view of their own compensation, physicians can adapt and create a fine medical system in which the clinical decisions are made by professionals. In such a system, physicians have the opportunity to become more efficient by managing care through teams rather than providing it all personally. A comforting factor is that there are so many patients that are underserved by the health care system that if all of them were brought into the system for care, all available physicians would be necessary. Thus, adapting does not have to mean lay-offs.

Incentives into Paradigm Shift

The progressive application of high-level incentives can result in a paradigm shift in service delivery under the right conditions within medical groups (Burns, Bazzoli, Dynan, & Wholey, 1997). Our argument is that given the historical background to provider compensation discussed previously, there are many constraints against such circumstances magically unfolding in the medical practice environment. However, the high-performing medical group will intentionally cultivate conditions wherein high-level incentives have a reasonable chance of succeeding; wherein innovative methods of motivating staff can produce a climate conducive to both individual and organizational goal accomplishment. Such a radical change in compensation and incentives does not just happen overnight. It requires careful planning and incremental implementation to overcome a long tradition in health care wherein physicians benefited at the expense of other staff and the health care organizations in which they practiced.

A progressive application of high-level incentives and its flow into paradigm shifts in service delivery are depicted in Figure 7.6. While truly high-performing medical groups might aspire to begin with a paradigm shift, experience suggests that progress is often paced at a slower rate. Little change can often add up to significant change. Small steps produce momentum, success and confidence, thereby allowing a higher rate of change. However, the ability to initiate large-scale shifts in service delivery should not be discounted. Figure 7.6 simply recognizes that the majority of medical groups will witness a

		Apply Cost-Savings Sharing		

Year	Service Cost	Savings Realized	Managed Care Cost	Staff	Group
1	$10,000,000	$2,500,000	$800,000	$800,000	$900,000
2	7,500,000	1,500,000	500,000	500,000	500,000
3	6,000,000	1,500,000	500,000	500,000	500,000

Achieves

Level of lowest feasible operating
cost in one service area

Expands
application

Apply cost-savings strategy to all
other cost-control areas

Achieves

Level of lowest feasible operating
cost in all service areas

Introduces

Paradigm shift in service delivery

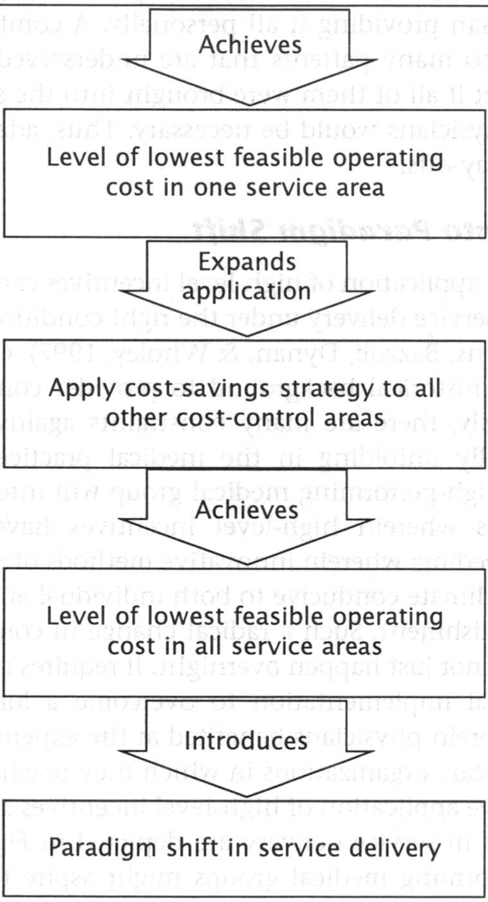

FIGURE 7.6   Progressive Application of High-Level Incentives

number of intervening steps before reaching the level of a paradigm shift that creates ingenious service breakthroughs.

A hypothetical medical group commits itself to delivering the right care at the right time with kindness, quality and low cost. To achieve this ambitious vision, the medical group's leaders understand that they must do something radical to encourage each staff member to control costs. A cost-sharing plan is discussed among a team of providers. For example, a urology group wants to reduce its cost of services to a managed care entity. By reducing the cost of service delivery to patients associated with the plan, the medical group will be able to offer the plan a lower contractual price for care coverage the following year. This ability to lower the price of care is particularly critical because a new urology group from a large, reputable medical group in a distant city has recently entered the market. This competitive threat calls for immediate action and demonstrable results in order to parlay the cost savings into a lower contract bid.

The medical group devises a cost-savings sharing program that includes every provider (physician and nonphysician) in the distribution of savings. In year 1, the projected service cost is $10 million. This figure is too high and will create a bid that is not competitive. The previous year, the same set of services were bid to the managed care plan at the same $10 million. It is unlikely that the managed care plan will continue this level of payment. It is seeking a cost reduction (mindful that it also wants the highest quality of care at the same time). It is also known that the plan is seriously attracted to the possibility of an alliance with the high-profile urology group, which has linkages to the network centered in the large city.

The first medical group must reduce its cost of care in order to deliver a lower bid. It projects that an 8 percent decrease in cost is necessary to retain the contract next year. Furthermore, it projects that an additional 10 percent total decrease in price must occur over the following two years in order to retain the managed care contract. In effect, it will have to reduce its contract price 18 percent over three years. This translates to a $1.8 million decrease in the price of the managed care contract.

The medical group is concerned but not desperate. The staff has been pilot testing a number of new strategies to enhance productivity, and it has reconfigured service delivery around teams. The staff is convinced it can lower the cost of service by 40 percent over three years—this represents an additional savings of 22 percent over the cost of the original managed care contract in year 1. How can the group of urologists share the cost savings to provide the incentives needed to ensure the cost reductions while simultaneously meeting the financial performance goals of the group and the reduced price goal for the managed care plan?

Figure 7.6 demonstrates the use of higher-level incentives through cost-savings allocation. In year 1, the group achieves $2.5 million in savings. This sum is split three ways—the staff and the group receive $800,000 and $900,000, respectively, to allocate and the remaining $800,000 is used to reduce the price of the managed care contract. The point of this illustration is that everyone benefits by introducing enlightened incentives. The managed care plan receives a lower price, staff has higher compensation for hard work and the medical group owners benefit from a higher return on investment.

The profile for the group in years 2 and 3 mimics year 1 but at a lower level. The urology group is only able to squeeze out an additional $1.5 million in savings within each year. However, the decreases are sufficient to motivate staff, to lower the price of services and to add to return on investment. Clearly, the key to success is the set of strategies used to reduce the cost of care while maintaining the quality of care. Prior chapters have described many strategies and tactics by which such savings can be realized. The challenge to medical groups is to devise similar strategies and tactics and then to carefully implement them.

Taking the Next Step

The urology group's clever use of incentive strategies to reduce costs and to apply high-level incentives is only the beginning of effective management. Having experienced first-hand the value of instilling high-level incentives, the medical group can apply the same approach to other areas. The result is a progressive application of high-level incentives to many areas. Having achieved the level of lowest feasible cost in one service area, the urology group is then motivated to apply the principle to other areas. If those applications are somewhat equivalent in results, the outcome for the urology group is to attain the lowest level of feasible operating cost in all service areas. At this point, the medical group has truly positioned itself as a distinctive competitor and a preferred provider. However, the scenario does not stop there because the medical group inhabits a very contentious, competitive environment. It cannot rest on its past accomplishments; it must attend to the threats presented by other providers. How can it respond under these circumstances?

Figure 7.6 suggests that, after successive attempts and victories at developing incremental cost-sharing solutions (for example, in years 1, 2 and 3), the medical group will eventually exhaust the opportunities and tactics for achieving the lowest feasible operating cost in all service areas. In effect, the easy methodologies for deriving cost savings are all considered and either discarded or applied. At this point, the group still has an answer to the issue of achieving cost savings—a paradigm shift. The group can move to another level of strategizing by reengineering service delivery processes. This implies being open to wholesale changes within care delivery.

The chain of improvements shown in Figure 7.6 represents incremental changes that progressively bring the medical group to a significant goal—the lowest feasible cost in all service areas. This successive incrementalism is planned and well orchestrated as far as getting most people to accept widespread change. By instilling smaller changes over a longer period of time, the same outcome is eventually achieved, albeit after a longer period of time.

This coordinated incrementalism can be avoided in the most progressive, transcendental groups. Rather than thinking about how incremental gains can be achieved, the leadership of the group can push for a radical, but reasoned, alteration in care delivery. This approach is often characterized as working smarter rather than harder or as reengineering of basic service or production processes. It is not analogous to continuous improvement efforts that seek to fine-tune processes over long periods.

In the final analysis, the progressive application of high-level incentives can lead to wonderful improvements in medical care delivery. Clinical environments are ripe for the use of such techniques. However, there remains for managers another approach that transcends even the implementation of very clever tactics. The managerial challenge is to remain sensitive to opportunities to apply these more comprehensive techniques while utilizing more incremental approaches until the environment presents an invitation for innovative solutions.

THE CONTRIBUTIONS OF VISIONARY LEADERS

Organizational visions are not enough to succeed in the tumultuous health care environment. They must be accompanied by visionary leaders. Who qualifies as a visionary leader? Is it just the top executive officer? Is it the board of directors? Or, is it the most senior physician who is able, through experience and insights gained over the years, to philosophize about the broad trends in health care and thus identify a critical path through the maze confronting a medical group? Perhaps the visionary leader is none of the above but rather a small cadre of doctors who have remained with the clinic through good times and bad. Still others might suggest that the visionary leader is an identifiable group of staff throughout the medical group that has a great idea about how the practice might be improved but senses that its fabulous idea might not be appreciated by others. A visionary leader might be an individual with the key for securing a large managed care contract.

All of the preceding people and groups could qualify for what we believe to be a visionary leader. There is a tendency to think that the top person in a medical group—whether physician executive or medical practice executive—is the person possessing the vision or is capable of articulating the dynamic, challenging and motivating vision of what a medical group should strive to become. On reflection, it should be clear that a vision does not necessarily have to spring from a single person. In fact, a top leader may be quite effective in getting others to express dynamic and passionate views of where an organization such as a medical group should be headed. This leader can then blend and temper these contributions into a single vision that is embraced by others and that comes to represent the very essence of the medical group.

Visionary leaders share a number of distinctive attributes that can be learned and, thus, implemented in the course of managing a medical group or other health care organization (McDaniel, 1997). Table 7.1 presents the distinctive attributes of visionary leaders along with explanations of how these attributes are applicable in medical groups. The challenge is to reflect on how leaders might internalize these attributes and incorporate them on a daily basis in their management activities and leadership roles (Shields, 1994). Vision-setting is an everyday task rather than some activity that a medical group member completes at the time of strategic planning. This thought is consistent with the growing

TABLE 7.1   The Attributes of Visionary Leaders

Distinctive Attributes of Visionary Leaders	*Applicability in Medical Groups*
1. *Encourage paradigm shifts:* If the service delivery process is working modestly or is fraught with barriers, visionary leaders will be willing to try something different.	1. Clinical care delivery has been bandaged and treated superficially instead of receiving appropriate surgery. Medical group reform will require revolution in operations rather than surface improvements.
2. *Anticipate dynamic conservatism:* Visionary leaders anticipate that people will try to maintain the status quo and use this anticipation to their advantage.	2. Clinicians tend to reach a high comfort level with standard practice procedures. They will go to great efforts to resist change.
3. *Set challenging but reachable visions:* Visionary leaders define concrete stretches of aspiration that can be substantially achieved within three to five years. The visions are probability-favorable.	3. Medical professionals are driven by the need to achieve. They can be intensely motivated if they are presented goals that make them stretch.
4. *Use visions as a guideline for decisions:* The vision clarifies criteria for determining how to allocate resources and what strategies to pursue.	4. Visions function as templates or criteria against which administrative and clinical decisions are weighed.
5. *Integrate others' visions:* Even the alternative vision of the most ardent nonsupporters must fit with or be explained within the overarching vision.	5. Physicians and other highly educated medical professionals tend to develop passionate beliefs about their practices and the organization in which they practice. These passionate beliefs must be recorded within the overarching vision.
6. *Replay the story:* Visionary leaders continually replay the story of their vision. The vision motivates people to embark on a quest of the reachable. The importance of this quest is affirmed repeatedly.	6. The vision as a story achieves clarity of understanding and a source of inspiration. It focuses attention on why people are in the medical group and how their personal effort will lead to something distinctive and important.
7. *Channel consensus:* Group processes are used to consistently build consensus and support for the vision.	7. Groups and teams are the fundamental architecture for reaching decisions and tackling problems. Group activities are driven by a view of the possible.

evidence that effective visions are vibrant operating principles that inform and mold the actions of medical group staff members.

Encourage Paradigm Shifts

More than any other distinctive characteristic, visionary leaders are noted for their ability to encourage creative thinking as an organizational asset. Perhaps the creative initiative is a new structure for the group (Korenchuk & Hord, 1996) or a shift to more satellite clinics (Harper, 1995). Whatever the initiative, visionary leaders emphasize creativity. They reinforce how important it is to think in creative and nontraditional ways about problems that medical groups face. **Visionary leaders have observed and experienced many times over how important it is to approach really tough problems from new perspectives.** They realize that innovation and change are very threatening, especially to those who stand to gain the most from not changing. Nonetheless, visionary leaders do not back off their commitment to resolve—rather than continue—difficult issues. They have the clarity of mind to know that incremental, band-aid solutions seldom get the job done. It is the brilliant concept that ultimately shifts the paradigm of thinking and allows fresh strategies to work their miracles.

This ability to encourage paradigm shifts has particular applicability for medical groups. The problem with the health care system is that it needs sweeping reform to resolve the issues that have made its expense intolerable. Medical groups reflect this dilemma when only the most marginal changes are accepted as a means to continue without true change. Specifically, clinical care delivery has been bandaged and treated superficially in the progressive efforts to rein in health care costs. The health care system needs surgery, not palliative remedies. The implication for medical groups is that a revolution in operations (that is, care delivery) rather than superficial improvements has become necessary.

It is unlikely that shallow, disjointed adjustments by medical groups to the health care environment will ever help them reach a state of transcendence. **Visionary leadership, however, could provide the means for medical groups to approach care delivery in exciting and viable, new ways that not only improve the health care cost picture, but that also enhance the quality of care (the ability to do the right thing at the right time with effectiveness, kindness, and low cost).**

Anticipate Dynamic Conservatism

Donald Schon (1971) introduced the concept of dynamic conservatism more than 25 years ago when he observed that organizations and systems will do everything in their power not to change. Instead, they present an atmosphere of frenzied activity in which little change is actually introduced. Their hyperactive machinations are simply a disguise for conservative entrenchment. **The more dynamic or frenzied the atmosphere or profile that an organization/system displays, the more conservative is the actual amount of change introduced, according to Schon's law.** The ultimate display of dynamic conservatism is to entrench even further and to solidify the status quo.

Visionary leaders anticipate dynamic conservatism. They recognize that medical group staff members will likely avoid changing if they are able. Physicians are notorious for their hesitation to alter the status quo. This built-in barrier to improving operations is a fact of life that visionary leaders not only anticipate, but relish, as a managerial challenge. The astute leader will view dynamic conservatism in a gaming sense. Before introducing a new concept, the leader will carefully identify the individuals who stand to be significantly affected by change. Visionary leaders will then answer how they can establish an incentive for staff to leave the status quo behind. Answers to this knotty problem will inevitably require a strong measure of paradigm shifting.

As Table 7.1 suggests, clinicians tend to reach extraordinarily high comfort levels given the status quo of the health care system. Physicians have especially been protected from many of the deleterious effects of health care reform even if they would not openly admit it. Despite the adoption of managed care throughout the health system, practicing medicine is still an envied and very attractive profession. Certainly, there has been some erosion in physician perquisites, but by and large, doctors enjoy enormous benefits not available to others. Consequently, physicians will go to great lengths to resist change. Visionary leaders anticipate this behavior and plan counteractive measures accordingly.

Set Challenging Visions

Visionary leaders are renowned for setting challenging but achievable visions. They want to make their organizations stretch while simultaneously ensuring that there is a high probability that the vision will be attained. For these reasons, visions should have a high favorable probability. If the vision is too lofty, it will be difficult to measure progress and, hence, provide sufficient immediate feedback that encourages further action toward the vision. In contrast, an easily achievable vision does not provide the motivation to staff to stretch toward something higher—a level of performance that distinguishes the medical group.

Medical groups should use the concept of setting challenging but achievable visions to their advantage in view of their constituents— physicians. It is readily apparent that physicians tend to be very motivated and goal oriented. If they were not, they would have encountered significant difficulty in making it through medical school. Medical professionals are driven by the need to achieve. It is an intrinsic reward for many physicians and nurses. They can be intensely motivated if they are presented goals that make them stretch. Thus, visionary leaders can assess the goal orientation of their colleagues and respond accordingly.

Visions as Guidelines for Decisions

One of the most useful characteristics of a vision is its ability to function as a guideline or framework for decision making. A vision essentially points the way for a medical group, and along with this direction, expresses indicators of where resources should be expended, which opportunities should be overlooked, who should be promoted and a host of other vital decisions. **In this respect, a vision becomes a very useful management tool as it clarifies criteria for determining how to allocate resources, which goals to establish and what strategies to pursue.**

Visionary leaders capitalize on this aspect of visions. In a medical group, the vision functions as a template or criterion against which administrative and clinical decisions are weighed. For example, the decision to add a nephrologist to a medical group can be answered partially by referring to the group's vision. Does the group wish to pursue specialty care (Barnett, 1996)? Does it wish to offer subspecialty care? How will the nephrology specialist fit within the ensemble of existing primary and specialty services? What programmatic areas will the nephrologist fulfill? How will the nephrologist help the medical group achieve distinction for a type of care? What resources are needed to support the nephrologist? The questions can continue, but the key point is that visionary leaders use a vision to answer these questions rather than dwelling on the often political issues that will be raised along with the concerns of medical staff expansion.

Integrate Others' Visions

Every medical group experiences it at one time or another. The truly unfortunate medical groups have a history of the problem. The most unfortunate groups are recognized for their inability to get along with one another. A contentious medical staff is one constraint that visionary leaders would just as soon do without. Nonetheless, it is perhaps the nature of physician groups that they do not always foster the best of interpersonal relations **Visionary leaders must be constantly cognizant that their group is comprised of brilliant professionals who are socialized to act and think independently.** Medical education places enormous value on decision making, especially autonomous decision making. Thus, visionary leaders can anticipate resistance to their group's vision. They should assume that at least some of the key medical staff will covertly (if not overtly) denigrate the vision (if not demonstrate outright resistance).

Recognizing that some professionals simply must challenge any forms of authority—as represented by the group's vision—provides an advantage to the visionary leader. He or she will attempt to integrate others' (particularly nonsupporters') visions, or portions thereof, within the final articulated, overarching vision. This approach recognizes that highly educated medical professionals tend to develop passionate beliefs about their practices and the organization with which they choose to practice. These passionate beliefs must be reconciled within the overarching vision.

Replay the Story

Table 7.1 indicates that visionary leaders are not hesitant to replay the story; that is, they continually tell the story of their vision. In this storytelling, they emphasize the wonderful goal that the organization will achieve. Visionary leaders tell the story of passion for achieving something great—something distinctive—that only this organization can possible achieve. The vision story is often rooted in significant accomplishments the organization has made in the past. Legendary heroes are remembered for their courage and ability to withstand tough times or to take on larger foes while coming out a winner. In many cases, the stories have been molded into myths that, over time, have made the players and the stakes larger than they truly were when the events unfolded. The stories especially tell of individual personal sacrifice that helped the organization succeed despite overwhelming odds.

Visionary leaders use these stories to motivate people toward inspired performance. The stories convey that the lofty aspirations of the organization were once thought impossible but, in actuality, were attainable. The link is made to the current vision as yet another chapter in the saga of the organization to overcome the forces. The visionary leader uses this allusion to a distinctive heritage to help staff members understand that they are part of a continuing history—something larger than the immediate moment and something more significant than any one person.

For medical groups, the vision as a story achieves clarity of understanding for group members. For example, a licensed practical nurse may understand the vision as story that enables her or him to better realize that the medical group is more interested in achieving something truly special—not just caring for one patient after another. To the physician, the vision should become the very reason for practicing medicine. The group has elevated its aspirations to a level befitting the practice of medicine. In short, the vision as a story focuses attention on why people are in the medical group and how their personal effort will lead to an outcome that is rare and precious.

Channel Consensus

Finally, Table 7.1 suggests that visionary leaders use visions to channel group consensus. If the vision is used repeatedly to focus discussions on resource allocations, problem resolutions and new goals to pursue, eventually the communication among group members will be channeled toward a similar, consistent belief in the desirable. Once medical group members are using the same language and the same frame of reference (that is, the vision), then it is more likely that consensus will form and a cohesiveness will develop within the group.

Care delivery groups and teams are the fundamental architecture for reaching decisions and tackling tough problems. Visionary leaders attempt to encourage staff members to address problems in teams so that the resulting consensus facilitates implementation of resolutions. Group activities are driven by a view (that is, a vision) of the possible rather than dwelling on a recognition of the difficult. The common vision coordinates and binds the mutual efforts of medical group members to resolve community problems and to assist in supporting problems that, although localized in specific work units in the group, nonetheless pose a potential threat to the entire group practice.

THE VISION-SUPPORTIVE CULTURE

Having examined the attributes of visionary leaders, it is appropriate to close with a few thoughts about building vision-supportive cultures. Medical groups that achieve the distinctive do not just happen to do so by luck. We believe that exemplary medical groups are carefully crafted to be better than the rest (Grandinetti, 1997). **The distinguishing factor in attaining the high-performing medical group is the visionary leader—one who fosters a vision-supportive culture.** These relationships are depicted in Figure 7.7.

The vision of a high-performing medical group is to (clinically speaking) deliver the right care at the right time with kindness to patients and with effective cost and high quality. However, as Figure 7.7 suggests, simply having an inspiring vision does not necessarily mean that it will materialize. Key strategies that address costs, productivity, medical manufacturing, patient-system relations, malpractice and quality improvement and organization/management must be implemented to achieve the vision. The implementation of these strategies is contingent on a vision-supportive culture. The vision-supportive culture, in turn, is nurtured by visionary leaders. Having already examined the strategies, it is time to examine the vision-supportive culture.

There must be vibrant collegial interaction within a medical group to make progress toward attaining an inspirational vision. Sidebar 7.3 describes one approach for building this culture. Such interaction pertains to groups of professionals—physicians, nurses, technicians, and ancillary support—as well as among all staff (Kralewski, Wingert & Barbouche, 1996). A vision-supportive culture should incorporate every person as an integral part of the effort to deliver distinctive services. Furthermore, the collegial interaction is more than just feeling good about each other and the medical group. It implies an energetic drive to cooperatively (or collaboratively) reach a challenging goal (Allcorn, 1995). Staff will show evidence of a deep

Vision of the Transcendent Medical Group
- Right thing
- Right time
- Kindness to patients
- Effective cost
- With quality

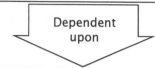

Dependent
upon

Vision-Supportive Culture
- Interaction is vibrant and collegial
- There is a willingness to experiment for the sake of improvement, and a commitment to a paradigm shift.
- Visions are used to guide decisions and orchestrate care delivery.
- The vision is a repeatedly shared story.
- Patients are actively included in the vision definition.

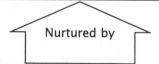

Nurtured by

Visionary Leaders
- A respected source (senior physician, board of directors, chief executive officer) articulates the essence of the vision
- Leadership of key physicians who fine-tune and polish the vision
- Management that acts in brilliant ways to define and enact strategies necessary to achieve the vision
- Staff that embraces the vision with zeal and commitment (or who move on to other organizations)

FIGURE 7.7 Nurturing a Vision-Supportive Culture

passion for the services the medical group delivers and great commitment for the vision it aspires to attain.

Second, a vision-supportive culture demonstrates willingness to experiment for the sake of improvement. For example, a medical group is pervasively committed to a paradigm shift in thinking about how services should be delivered. Thus, the same old approaches are not an answer emanating from a vision-supportive culture. Physicians, nurses, administrators, and other staff are driven to improve service delivery—even if it means altering the status quo, which may have received previous acclaim for excellence. Staff thinks in terms of how to make service delivery better than it has been even if there is no overt pressure to change. The high-performing medical group seeks innovations to remain at the forefront of the field.

Vision-supportive cultures are able to focus squarely on their target—a distinctive vision. This is a third characteristic of a vision-supportive culture. Visions are used as guidelines for decision making. Thus, at both the operational and strategic levels, the vision serves as a framework for decisions and resource allocations. The vision provides a conceptual framework from which problems can be addressed. The end result is a methodical reaffirmation of the vision and belief in the vision by all staff members.

Finally, Figure 7.7 suggests that a vision-supportive culture depends on actively involving patients and other stakeholders within the definition of a medical group's vision (Fottler, Blair, Rotarius & Youngblood, 1996). Astute medical groups want as much patient buy-in to the mission as possible. Therefore, they should incorporate their constituents into the vision-setting and vision-redefinition processes to the greatest extent possible. Clearly, the number of constituents any medical group possesses is quite large and precludes a broad, democratic process. Nonetheless, it is feasible to approximate broad patient (and other constituent) involvement. For example, managed care plan representatives, along with a few select patient representatives, may provide the kind of insights that elevate the medical group's vision because of external input.

Visionary Leaders

The visionary-supportive culture does not just suddenly materialize or otherwise evolve from an inexplicable source. Hard work on the part of visionary leaders nurtures the vision-supportive culture and, in the

SIDEBAR 7.3
Discerning a Medical Group's Culture

Reynolds (1986) has suggested that organization cultures can be characterized according to 12 dimensions:

1. External emphasis on customers versus internal activities emphasis;
2. Emphasis on completing tasks versus the social needs of staff;
3. Risk aversion in seeking innovation versus risk taking for new opportunities;
4. Toleration of individuality versus desire for conformity;
5. Individual versus collective decision making;
6. Centralized versus decentralized decision making;
7. Tendency for the organization to innovate versus remain stable;
8. Degree to which cooperation is emphasized over competition;
9. Degree of complexity of the organization versus efforts to keep things simple;
10. Emphasis on detailed rules versus flexibility;
11. Loyalty to the organization versus other organizations; and
12. Degree of communicated knowledge of organizational expectations.

Not every culture is expected to emphasize all of these dimensions. Rather, an organizational culture achieves its distinctiveness by embracing several of these cultural dimensions and institutionalizing them as unique properties of what that particular organization means.

Kralewski, Wingert and Barbouche (1996) operationalized these dimensions in a survey instrument designed to assess the organizational culture of medical groups. Their instrument was refined through testing on 100 clinics in the Minneapolis/St. Paul metropolitan area. Reynolds's 12 dimensions were reduced to nine prevailing dimensions within the medical groups, including:

1. Innovativeness and risk taking;
2. Group solidarity;
3. Cost-effectiveness orientation;
4. Organizational formality;
5. Method of cost control;

continued

6. Centralization of decision making;

7. Entrepreneurism;

8. Physician's individuality; and

9. Visibility of costs.

This instrument offers one approach to measuring the congruency of medical group members' views of their organizational culture.

Kralewski, Wingert and Barbouche then applied the instrument to two different groups that they believed reflected decidedly different organization culture orientations. Their predictions held true as shown by the following cultural dimensions emphasized by each medical group:

Group A	*Group B*
Method of cost control	Innovativeness and risk taking
Centralization of decision making	Group solidarity
Entrepreneurism	Cost-effectiveness orientation
Physician individuality	Organizational formality
Visibility of costs	

The notable implication of this study is that every group possesses a distinctive culture. To the extent that medical group members (for example, physicians and staff) align themselves with a group that reflects the cultural dimensions that they value, the culture should improve and become more powerful. Medical groups that are not able to instill a common culture are susceptible to inferior performance as members are distracted by the political interplay to reach a dominant culture.

Source: Adapted from J. K. Kralewski, T. D. Wingert, & M. H. Barbouche. (1996). Assessing the culture of medical group practices. *Medical Care, 34*(5), 377–388.

---

final analysis, creates the high-performing medical group. Figure 7.7 indicates that visionary leaders who nurture the culture may be found from a wide variety of professionals. Typically, a respected source articulates the vision that the culture attempts to operationalize. The respected source may be a senior physician, the board of directors or the chief executive officer. Regardless of who the source is, the common denominator of the visionary leader is the ability to carefully articulate a first-rate vision.

Visionary leaders may involve key physicians who fine-tune, polish or hone the vision. Once a straw vision statement is crafted, it requires improvement and distillation. The key physicians in the medical group are extremely important in this regard. They will generally support the attempt to stretch the reach of the group, but they will also keep the extent of the stretch within bounds, capabilities and resources.

Visionary leaders may include management staff who act in brilliant ways to define and implement strategies necessary to achieve the vision. The best medical group vision statement in the world is worthless unless purposeful and successful action toward its attainment is initiated. Medical practice executives have substantial responsibility to ensure that a plan of action is delineated and progressively implemented in order to attain the vision.

Finally, but just as important as other leaders depicted in Figure 7.7, staff members who embrace the vision with zeal and commitment function as vision heroes. They are the ones who operationalize the strategies. They are the ones who make certain that the right thing is done at the right time. They determine whether care is delivered with great kindness at low cost and high quality. And, if by chance a medical group has staff members who cannot internalize this intense feeling for the group's vision, then they best move to another competitor. **The exceptional—high-performing—medical group attempts to make certain that every staff member is a champion for achieving the best that medical groups can become—a leader in the effort to reform the health care system.**

APPLICATIONS FOR MANAGERS

Enlightened organizational and visionary management is one of the most important distinguishing differences between the typical medical group that is slowly making its contribution in a rather pedestrian way and the medical group that everyone looks up to with great admiration. There is nothing wrong with being a status quo medical group in favorable times or in a propitious setting, but things seldom remain the same, and what was once a wonderfully supportive environment can rapidly change into a highly threatening quagmire. The comfortable setting and casual attitude of the group intersect with a world turned upside down. Without practical experience in managing new constraints or a conceptual model for surviving the disastrous forces, the future grows dim.

Medical practice executives have a distinct choice when it comes to how they manage the strategic response of their organization. They can sit back and wait for things to happen, or they can aggressively introduce change. Whether they want it to be this way or not, the sad truth is that almost no one in the health care field has the luxury of waiting to see what will develop next. A wait-and-see attitude is a prerequisite for hanging out a for-sale sign.

Enlightened organization and management—the fortitude to introduce inspiring visions, to cultivate distinctive competencies, to introduce brilliant organizational advancements or to instill high-level incentives—costs very little. These efforts are well within the capability of every group if staff members will pull together as a team and embrace an attitude that innovation leads to better individual and organizational well-being.

REFERENCES

Allcorn, S. (1995, September/October). The group dynamics of medical practices. *MGM Journal*, 88–100.

Argysis, C., & Schon, D. (1978). *Organizational learning: A theory of action perspective.* Reading, MA: Addison-Wesley.

Barnett, A. A. (1996, October 28). Is there a future in single specialty groups? *Medical Economics*, 58–68.

Bart, C. K., & Tabone, J. C. (1999, Summer). Mission statement content and hospital performance in the Canadian not-for-profit health care sector. *Health Care Management Review, 24*(3), 18–29.

Bart, C. K., & Tabone, J. C. (1998). Mission statement rationales and organizational alignment in the not-for-profit health care sector. *Health Care Management Review, 23*(4), 54–69.

Burns, L. A. (1996). Physicians and group practice: Balancing autonomy with market reality. *Journal of Ability Care Management, 19*(3), 1–15.

Burns, L. R., Bazzoli, G. J., Dynan, L., & Wholey, D. R. (1997). Managed care, market stages, and integrated delivery systems: Is there a relationship? *Health Affairs, 16*(6), 204–218.

Derrick, F. W. & Scott, C. E. (1995, Summer). National health insurance: lessons from the United States experiment. *Health Care Management Review, 20*(3): 55–63.

Devers, K. J., Shortell, S. M., Gillies, R. R., Anderson, D. A., Mitchell, J. B., & Morgan Erickson, K. L. (1994). Implementing organized delivery systems: An integration scorecard. *Health Care Management Review, 19*(3), 7–20.

Fgdahl, R. H., & Taft, C. H. (1986). Sounding Board: Financial incentives to physicians. *New England Journal of Medicine, 23*(5), 461–483.

Evolution in group practice management. (1998, January/February). *MGM Journal*, 72–78.

Fottler, M. D., Blair, J. D., Rotarius, T. M., & Youngblood, M. R. (1996, May/June). Strategic choices for medical group practices. *MGM Journal,* 32–50.

Grandinetti, D. A. (1997, April 7). What it takes for big groups to succeed. *Medical Economics,* 87–116.

Harper, T. F. (1995, September 11). Satellites: What groups have learned the hard way. *Medical Economics,* 70–80.

Herbert, M. E. (1997, March/April). A for-profit health plan's experience and strategy. *Health Affairs,* 121–124.

Hill, J., & Mullen, P. (1996, January). Exploring practice management options. *Healthcare Financial Management,* 22–23.

Kertesz, L. (1998, April 13). Partnering with PSOs. *Modern Healthcare,* 40–41.

Korenchuk, K. M. & Hord, J. M. (1996). Managed care plans and the organizational arrangements with group practices. *Journal of Ambulatory Care Management, 19*(4), 11–17.

Kralewski, J. E., Rich, E. C., Bernhardt, T., Dowd, B., Feldman, R., & Johnson, C. (1998). The organizational structure of medical group practices in a managed care environment. *Health Care Management Review, 23*(21), 76–96.

Kralewski, J. E., Wingert, T. D., & Barbouche, M. H. (1996). Assessing the culture of medical group practices. *Medical Care, 34*(5), 377–388.

Kwon, S. (1996). Structure of financial incentive systems for providers in managed care plans. Medical Care Research and Review, 53(2), 149–161.

Larwood, L., Falbe, C. M., Kriger, M. P., & Miesing, P. (1995, June). Structure and the meaning of organizational vision. *Academy of Management Journal, 38*(3), 740–769.

Lowes, R. (1996, December 23). How a group's personality affects its members. *Medical Economics,* 35–47.

Magnus, S. A. (1999). Physicians' financial incentives in five dimensions. *Health Care Management Review, 24*(1), 45–56.

McDaniel, R. R. (1997). Strategic leadership: A view from quantum and chaos theories. *Health Care Management Review, 22*(1), 21–37.

Meighan, S. S. (1995). Where have all the primary care physicians gone? *Health Care Management Review, 20*(3), 64–67.

Mintzberg, H. (1997). Toward healthier hospitals. *Health Care Management Review, 22*(4), 9–18.

Reynolds, P. D. (1986). Organizational culture as related to industry, position and performance: A preliminary report. *Journal of Management Studies, 23,* 333.

Robinson, J. C. (1996). The dynamics and limits of corporate growth in health care. *Health Affairs, 15*(2), 155–169.

Schon, D. (1971). *Beyond the stable state.* New York: Random House.

Shields, M. C. (1994, September/October). The physician-administrator team revisited. *MGM Journal, 41*(5): 10, 110.

Shortell, S. M., Devers, K. J., Gillies, R. R., Anderson, D. A., Mitchell, J. B., & Erickson, K. L. (1994, Summer). Implementing organized delivery systems: an integration scorecard. *Health Care Management Review, 19*(3): 7–20.

Stuart, M. E., & Weinrich, M. (1998). Beyond managing Medicaid costs: Restructuring care. *The Milbank Quarterly, 76*(2), 251–280.

Unland, J. J. (1995). The evolution of physician-directed managed care. *Journal of Health Care Finance, 22*(2), 42–56.

Weil, T. P. (1995, March/April). Why is medical group management now so contentious? *MGM Journal,* 60–72.